MW00649947

IF YOU OR A LOVED ONE HAS EAR, ALLERGY PROBLEMS, YOU MUST READ THIS BOOK! This revolutionary book brings help and hope to adults and children afflicted by chronic diseases of the ears, sinuses, or respiratory tract. Dr. David S. Hurst, MD, PhD, is a leading researcher in the field of allergic ear disease. His book is candid, complete, and gives a no holds barred account of research breakthroughs and treatment options in this very controversial field.

Dr. Hurst exposes the fatal flaws in some diagnostic tests, and outlines how to diagnose and effectively treat even the most difficult cases. Here is a comprehensive summary of our current knowledge, with a discussion of what actually works. The book is a self-teaching guide that contains all the essential facts to enable you to know when you are getting treatment that works.

– Bruce R. Gordon, M.D., F.A.C.S.
Department of Laryngology & Otology, Harvard Medical School
Past President, American Academy of Otolaryngic Allergy

✂

In spite of years of training, many medical specialists merely treat otitis rather than finding and eliminating the cause. In this book, *Freedom from Chronic Ear Infections,* a dedicated, knowledgeable ear specialist approaches recurrent medical problems in the ears by asking "Why?" He puts it all together and, in a neat package, explains how it happens and what you need to do in order to prevent recurrent fluid behind the eardrums along with the resulting hearing loss. Many who read this book will quickly (in a very few weeks) recognize how they can resolve their own child's recurrent ear disease, often all on their own. Sit down in a comfy chair, relax, and read the answers you have been asking for, perhaps for years. Your child deserves a life without ear infections and to have optimum hearing.

– Doris J. Rapp, M.D.
Board Certified in Pediatrics (Emeritus) at SUNYAB
Author of *Our Toxic World: A Wake-Up Call*
www.drrapp.com

CR

Finally, physicians and parents alike have a compendium loaded with factual information to assess the role allergy plays in the causes and treatment of childhood middle ear problems.   There are many factors that contribute to the cause of chronic ear infections in children and for a long time no one had really known how much allergy is a cause of ear infections. Therefore, physicians and parents of children who are trying to find the best way to treat children afflicted with ear infections, persistent middle ear fluid, or both, have had difficulty knowing when and how to utilize allergy management in the treatment of childhood middle ear problems. Dr. David Hurst has devoted much of his professional career to scientifically investigating these issues and, thankfully, his treatise *Freedom from Ear Infections* contains all the information anyone would need. This manuscript is exhaustive and comprehensive – it is thoughtful and well written. Certainly we need to get this information out to all who care for children.

– Kenneth M. Grundfast, M.D., F.A.C.S.
Chair of Otolaryngology, Boston University School of Medicine.
Past President of the American Society of Pediatric Otolaryngology
Past Vice President of the American Academy of
Otolaryngology-Head and Neck Surgery
Chair, Department of Otolaryngology-Head and Neck Surgery,
Boston University School of Medicine

CR

Dr. David Hurst is a true and relentless scientist, fiercely loyal to observation of natural phenomena in his field. He brings his formidable energy and talent to investigate a crucial problem long shrouded in mystery: the role of allergy in middle ear disease. Children needlessly receive extended antibiotic regimens or are treated with ear tubes that do not address the real problems. This book is the culmination of decades of Dr. Hurst's diligent and untiring work. In my view, it resolves the central question in middle ear pathology completely. I fervently hope it will receive wide readership which it richly deserves. I fervently hope all physicians who care for children will read Dr. Hurst's book.

– Majid Ali, MD, F.R.C.S.
Professor of Medicine, Emeritus, Capital University,
Washington, D.C.

CR

FREEDOM FROM
CHRONIC EAR INFECTIONS

The Role of Allergies and the Way to a Cure

*A book designed to help you understand
how allergy leads to chronic middle ear disease,
asthma, and sinusitis, and how to cure them.*

David S. Hurst, M.D., Ph.D.

BACK CHANNEL PRESS
- PORTSMOUTH, NH -

FREEDOM FROM
CHRONIC EAR INFECTIONS
The Role of Allergies and the Way to a Cure
Copyright © 2011 by David Hurst
ISBN 13: 978-1-934582-37-4
Library of Congress PCN 2011903179

BACK CHANNEL PRESS
170 Mechanic Street
Portsmouth, NH 03801
www.backchannelpress.com

Printed in the United States of America

Design and layout by Nancy W. Grossman

Cover photo © Copyright 2011 Roy Tennant, FreeLargePhotos.com

The information in this book is intended for general education purposes only and should not be relied upon as a substitute for professional and/or medical advice. If you have any specific questions about any medical matter you should consult your doctor or other professional healthcare provider. You should never delay seeking medical advice, disregard medical advice, or discontinue medical treatment because of information contained herein.

Copyright permissions:

Table I, page 142, adapted from: Hurst DS: The middle ear: The inflammatory response in children with otitis media with effusion and the impact of atopy. Clinical and histochemical studies., in Comprehensive Summaries of Uppsala Dissertations from the Faculty of Medicine, Dept of Immunology and Clinical Chemistry #978. Uppsala, Sweden: Uppsala University, Sweden, 2000, p 14, with permission.

Tables II and III, pages 143 and 144, reprinted from: Hurst DS. Efficacy of allergy immunotherapy as a treatment for patients with chronic otitis media with effusion. *Int J Pediatr Otorhinolaryngol.* Aug 2008;72(8):1215-1223., with permission from Elsevier.

Figures 16-19 Adapted with permission from figure 2 in: *Arch Otolaryngol Head Neck Surg.* May 2002;128(5):564, copyright 2002; American Medical Association, all rights reserved.

This book is dedicated to my wife Melissa, a better physician and immunologist than I could ever be, who has provided her love, unreserved support and guidance; and to my mother Lynn who encouraged me to finish whatever project I had engaged and who in the end was there but did not know.

ACKNOWLEDGEMENTS

My thanks first to my patients for showing the way by asking the basic question: "Why?" and for teaching me to listen and for entrusting to me their care. Thanks also to my mentor Dr. Per Venge who is a man with more integrity than any I have ever known; and to my many other teachers among whom in particular were Dr. Werner Chasin for giving me a chance as a resident and teaching that "Otolaryngology is half surgery and half medicine," Dr. Collin Karmody who taught me the microanatomy of the middle ear, Dr. Charles Bluestone who demanded no less than excellence and Dr. Alan McDaniels who encouraged me to "go for it." My thanks also to Gay Grant for her editing skills and for believing in the concept these past six years.

The opinions expressed in this book are solely my own and are not endorsed by any other physician, society, medical academy or organization.

"The imposition of orthodoxy (goes) hand-in-hand with a stifling of any form of independent reasoning."
– Charles Freeman: *The closing of the Western mind: the rise of faith and the fall of reason.* London, 2002.

"Advocates of evidence based medicine have criticized the adoption of interventions evaluated by using only observational data. We think that everyone may benefit if the most radical protagonists of evidence based medicine organized and participated in a double-blind, randomized, placebo-controlled, crossover trial of the parachute."
– Parachute use to prevent death and major trauma related to gravitational challenge: systematic review of randomized controlled trials. Gordon Smith, Jill Pell: *British Medical Journal* 2003; 327:1459 – 61.

« CONTENTS »

      A technical chapter for doctors and others who
      wish to read further and judge the scientific
      evidence for themselves.

« FIGURES »

« PREFACE »

WHY AND HOW I BECAME INTERESTED IN CHILDREN WITH CHRONIC EAR DISEASE

"Doctor, my child always has fluid in his ears!
Do you think he might have allergies?"

I am writing to you, parents and patients, to suggest that you become your own advocates. I have run out of patience for my fellow physicians who turn a deaf ear to the misery of young children with chronic middle ear fluid, thus sentencing them to years of hearing loss, delayed speech and learning disabilities. All of this suffering is completely reversible — better still, prevented in the first place. So this book is for you, the parent of a child — or the child who has become an adult him/herself — who continues to struggle with chronic middle ear fluid.

From reading this book, you will understand the underlying cause of chronic middle ear fluid and its risk factors. You will learn why only certain people have recurrent ear fluid, what allergies are, and how allergies affect the middle ear. Most important, you will learn what you can do to get your ears, or your child's ears, to stay normal — with 90 percent certainty.

Although this book is for people with chronic middle ear disease, the same concepts will benefit those of you who have chronic sinus disease or asthma, as 80% of these are likewise due to allergies. It is written to provide a basic primer for "allergy treatment for dummies," covering most aspects of allergy to help in your understanding of many allergy concepts including testing and treatment options for allergy to inhalants, molds and foods.

It is not unrealistic to expect that your ears or your child's ears should be "normal." In this book I will show that *allergy* is the cause of most chronic middle ear fluid, and that aggressive use of standardized allergy management can solve the problem. You will learn why ears develop chronic fluid and how this can be prevented. I will also explain that chronic middle ear disease and acute ear infections are two entirely different diseases, even though many doctors wrongly treat them the same way. I will explain why many children with chronic ear disease also have a runny nose or asthma — as all are manifestations of allergic disease. We now know that the middle ear behaves like the rest of the upper airway — sinuses, nose, and lungs — and what has been learned about the allergic response in these areas may be applied to the study of the ear to help us understand chronic middle ear disease. I and dozens of other physicians around the world base this knowledge on years of clinical practice and positive patient results confirmed by scientific investigation.

I found that thirty years as an ear, nose, and throat (ENT) surgeon in a solo rural practice is a humbling experience. All of one's failures return and serve as constant reminders of the fallibility of one's medical care for patients with chronic middle ear disease. My frustration with the lack of resolution of my patients' ear disease, the recurrence of their middle ear fluid, the need to repeatedly reinsert ear tubes, and the observation that many patients had multiple allergic symptoms led me to question whether allergy was contributing to their ear disease.

This hunch was confirmed by my clinical observation. When the allergies of my patients with chronic middle ear disease were addressed, they were also suddenly able to control their ear disease, even after years of failure with other treatments. As a clinician, I knew this was not mere chance, that there must be a scientific explanation. Review of the medical literature yields sporadic reports of similar successful allergy management of chronic fluid in the ears by others over the past 70 years. *Only in the past 15 years do we now have the science to explain how allergies are responsible for chronic middle ear fluid. We also have effective treatments so that millions of children and adults are not consigned to the misery of living with chronic middle ear disease.*

MY DISCOVERY

In the first ten years of my practice as an ear, nose and throat surgeon, I thought I had all the answers and could "cure" these problem ears by putting in "aeration tubes." After all, that is what all the courses at the academy meetings told us to do. The failures, we were taught, would only be cured by radical mastoid ear surgery, even though that would result in permanent hearing loss. Ear tubes are intended not so much to drain the fluid but to provide a way for air to get into the ear and dry things up. Yet some patients kept coming back for their third, fourth, and even fifth set of tubes. Something was clearly not working, but I noticed a pattern: many of these patients also had allergies. Some had continual runny noses and/or asthma. So I did my own clinical study.

I offered twenty patients in need of a third set of tubes a choice to either replace their tubes or try allergy treatment. All twenty patients were tested and found to be allergic by standard testing methods. Three chose no treatment and their ears remained full of fluid. In six patients whose allergies were treated for a time, the fluid cleared, but as soon as they quit their allergy shots or they ate the foods that made them congested, their ears filled up again, so I judged the treatment to have failed. Eleven maintained their allergy treatment for a full three years and remained free of middle ear fluid.

The results were clear after observing all twenty of these patients for three years. All eleven who remained on treatment were free of fluid in their middle ears; all nine who refused or stopped treatment had recurrence of their middle ear fluid. This study was my first published paper in a medical journal[1] and was the first report in the medical literature in years showing that allergy management had an effect on curing middle ear fluid. It is still quoted today. This study also led me to search for some marker of allergy in the middle ear of patients with persistent fluid in their ears.

It seemed to me that if we could understand the WHY, then we would know better WHAT to do.

In 1992, I attended an American Academy of Otolaryngic Allergy conference. The guest speaker, Dr. Per Venge of Sweden, spoke about the highly technical aspects of a little blood cell — the eosinophil — and its importance in the allergy reaction. After a long half hour with the lights out and lots of slides with little purple- and pink-colored cells, Dr. Venge concluded by suggesting that this eosinophil cell could serve as a marker in allergic inflammation as it affects all human tissue — brain, lung, joints, etc. It seems that this little cell leaves behind a marker that is only found in allergic reactions. I wondered if this could be the explanation on a cellular level for the connection between allergy and chronic middle ear fluid.

At lunch I made it a point to sit at Dr. Venge's table, and the first thing I asked him was: "Is this eosinophil cell in the middle ear?" He said he didn't know! I suggested that since he was the expert, with access to a lab in a hospital with 4,000 patient beds, perhaps he could find out. "You send me some ear fluid," he replied, "and then we will find out."

That fateful conversation launched me on twelve years of research. Dr. Venge became my mentor and eventually sponsored my successful defense of my Ph.D. dissertation on this topic.

This was an exciting time in the field of immunology, as technology allowed the investigation of cellular functions and component chemicals and enzymes responsible for the allergic mechanisms throughout the body. I have since published eighteen papers in the most influential medical journals in Europe and the United States confirming the presence of these components within the middle ear fluid of hundreds of patients. And that little eosinophil that Dr. Venge was talking about has been confirmed in middle ear fluid — at levels 300 times that seen in the lungs of severe asthmatics!

Unfortunately, even though we now have this scientific proof, most physicians still have not adopted this information; they still do not evaluate children with chronic ear fluid for allergies. At medical meetings, despite the best scientific evidence, there are allergists and ENT surgeons, including those in academia, who refuse to "believe" that allergy has anything to do with middle ear disease. Not surprising: After all, it took physicians 150 years to stop using leeches for the treatment of pneumonia despite published proof in 1730 that leeches had no beneficial effect on the disease!

A CLASSIC EXAMPLE OF HOW UNDIAGNOSED ALLERGY LEADS TO A LIFE OF DISASTROUS RESULTS

Albert, age 24

Albert's impossible case was presented at a "Grand Rounds" meeting by the chairman of a prestigious Boston teaching hospital. Albert had intermittent middle ear infections with persistent fluid since age 6. He had tubes placed twice. The third time larger "permanent tubes" were placed.

Albert's ears continued to drain pus intermittently from these tubes and he developed a secondary fungal infection. The tubes were removed. The eardrums were left with perforations because of the larger "permanent" tubes. Now both perforations drained intermittently. The only thing that the university hospitals could offer him was surgery.

Bilateral mastoidectmies were done which removed the bone that surrounded the middle ear and his eardrums were replaced. This left him with a permanent 30 to 40% hearing loss in each ear. Now both mastoid cavities are draining.

What was this poor fellow to do? Over 120 otolaryngologists were sitting in the room when the chairman asked if there were any suggestions. And so I raised my hand and asked: "What was his allergy status?" Well, he said:

Albert's allergy status was unknown!

The best of the university's best was certainly not good enough.

It amazes me how brilliant men and women who, during medical school and residency, were always questioning and whose brains were like sponges soaking up all the latest information, suddenly allow their brains to snap shut on graduation day. Now they know it all. Nothing new gets in. They didn't learn it before, therefore it must not be. These colleagues tell me, "I just don't believe it." I reply that parents and patients do not care about their physician's medical "beliefs" any more than they care about their religious beliefs; they just want their ears or their children's ears to be healed.

This book contains critical information for parents of young children, as well as adults who have long suffered with chronic middle ear disease. Four million children a year in the United States endure chronic fluid in their middle ears, resulting in hearing loss and delayed speech. *Tragically, children with hearing loss caused by chronic middle ear disease constitute the largest group of people with a reversible learning disorder in the world — a group that is generally ignored by pediatricians, ENT surgeons, and allergists.*

Sometimes in this book I will address you as the parent of a child with chronic middle ear fluid, and at other times I will slip into talking directly to you as a patient with fluid in your own ears. On occasion I will insert a letter sent as a question or comment to my Web page (www.earallergy.com). At other times I will present cases from my own patient files. When you finish this book you will understand why you continue to have fluid in your ears and how to prevent it. And your child does not need to spend the rest of his or her life on antibiotics that don't work. Nor should they, with rare exceptions, require repeated replacement of their ear tubes. Chronic middle ear fluid is common and treatable. Your child deserves "normal" ears, and with present medical knowledge you should settle for nothing less.

If you or your child is:

1. the person whose fluid persists for over two months;
2. the child or adult who has had more than one set of ear tubes;
3. the child who has tubes which continually drain;
4. the person with a hole in an eardrum which drains; and/or
5. the child who has failed their school hearing test and has no no history of ear infections —

— then this book is for you.

M.B., age 1

Hello,

I visited your webste, EARALLERGY.COM (among others) when my 1-year-old son was having recurring ear infections. He had tubes put in and this put a temporary end to a string of 8-10 ear infections. Six months later, he began to have them again, and hence my research. We were convinced that he might be suffering from an allergy, and so we removed milk from his diet, and took care of pillows and carpets in his room. He has remained infection free for over 8 months now, and the tubes which have long since fallen out are no longer needed.

Unfortunately for the patient, middle ear disease falls between the cracks of two medical subspecialties. Chronic middle ear fluid is usually treated by ENT surgeons (otolaryngologists), while allergies are usually treated by allergists or immunologists. Chronic middle ear fluid is ignored by both medical specialties because few of their members understand both ears *and* allergies.

Most ENT surgeons know little about allergy and almost no immunology. Furthermore, these specialists are concerned with bigger fish — like mastoid surgery, head and neck cancer, and putting in ear tubes. Their colleagues, the immunologists, focus on treating kids with life-threatening asthma or AIDS. Many of these specialists simply can't be bothered with tots with snotty noses — who also happen to have chronic ear disease.

In fact, most allergists or immunologists really do not know how to look at a middle ear correctly. ENT surgeons are specially trained to do so. You can see that for yourself because the allergist or pediatrician seldom uses what kids call "that little rubber bulb thing" on the ear instrument (called an otoscope) when they look in your child's ear. Without it the doctor can never know if there is fluid in the ear. Conversely, the allergist understands all the underlying mechanisms of allergy, which most ENT surgeons do not, but they never apply that knowledge to middle ear disease. (As some would say, "Well, ain't that odd?")

ENT surgeons are very interested in ears with chronic fluid, and even hold major international conferences on the topic. Yet few of them understand the immunologic mechanisms and effects of allergy even though one of their major concerns is the patient with chronic sinusitis (80 percent of whom have allergies). Fewer than one-tenth of all general ENT surgeons have taken the additional training required to be certified as an "ENT Allergist" by the American Academy of Otolaryngic Allergy (AAOA) or the Pan American Allergy Society (PAAS).

In terms of research, chronic otitis (the medical name for middle ear disease) is an orphan disease. Of over 10,570 articles published from 2001–2006 in the two major allergy journals (*Allergy* and *Journal of Allergy and Clinical Immunology*) and three major ENT journals (*Otolaryngology, Head and Neck Surgery*; *Laryngoscope*; and *Annals of Otolaryngology*), only sixteen articles were about allergy and middle ear disease. Funding from the pharmaceutical industry — which makes and markets antihistamines and antibiotics — drives research in ENT and allergy. It is not surprising then that these are the topics most often researched and written about in ENT and allergy medical journals.

In an effort to provide information on this subject for the public, I first created a Web site: www.earallergy.com. When I found myself spending an hour each evening answering patient questions, I thought perhaps a book would better serve the public. So I have chosen to turn directly to you, patients and parents who are frustrated with ineffective treatments for chronic middle ear fluid. Your drive to educate yourselves will empower you to find a physician who does have an interest in this disease — and there are hundreds of certified ENT allergists who can help you. Unfortunately, these few hundred can get lost in a sea of 7,000 ENT surgeons and 3,000 general allergists who practice in the United States, and who, in general, will not address the underlying cause of this fluid in the ears — *allergies.*

Parents want their children to stop having "ear infections" and maintain normal hearing. In this day of the Internet, information is power. In this book I will explain why not all allergy testing and all immunotherapy is the same. Once you have read and understood this little book, you will be armed with powerful information to bring your ears or your child's ears back to "normal" through the right course of testing, treatment, and follow-up with the right medical specialists. With the right information, you can bypass those in the medical establishment with entrenched "beliefs," and find a doctor with the knowledge to help you or your child. You can understand, question, and judge the quality and practicality of the information you obtain from any source, including my book. You can decide for yourself what is useful, and who is interested in helping you.

The World Wide Web allows you to seek the latest medical information in a way never before possible. This book will give you important background with which to evaluate the mass of information you may find on the Web. My Web page, www.earallergy.com, provides up-to-date information to accompany this book. Use the power of information wisely and your child *can* have "normal" ears.

You and your child have the RIGHT to effective treatment. No child with chronic middle ear fluid should be consigned to a lifetime of hearing loss and learning disabilities when it is now within our power to prevent or treat this condition.

« INTRODUCTION »

FINDING THE ALLERGY/CHRONIC MIDDLE EAR FLUID CONNECTION

Physicians call persistent fluid in the ear "otitis media with effusion," or OME. This condition is the major form of chronic relapsing inflammatory disease of the middle ear. In this book, I call this "chronic middle ear fluid." Chronic middle ear fluid is the most common medical diagnosis for children under 15 years old. The presence of chronic middle ear fluid may cause permanent damage, with scarring in the middle ear. Children with hearing loss secondary to OME constitute the largest group of people in the world with a reversible learning disorder. It is a disease of immense social and financial impact among families of young children, accounting for more than sixteen million office visits a year, at an annual cost of over $4 billion (2003 dollars) in the United States alone.[2] Seventeen percent of patients with an initial acute ear infection develop chronic middle ear fluid which persists at least twelve weeks or more after diagnosis, despite appropriate therapy.

The role of allergy in chronic middle ear disease is controversial. For seventy years our concept of the etiology of this disease had been founded on clinical observation alone. A simple explanation for the cause of chronic middle ear fluid had not emerged. New evidence from the fields of cellular biology and immunology now explain the basics of allergic reactions, and allow us to more accurately diagnose allergies and understand the allergic contribution to chronic inflammatory disease. Today we understand why some people genetically are more prone to ear infections than others. We also understand what triggers an ear to go from a simple infection to developing chronic fluid. Armed with this knowledge, we can treat the "why it happens."

UNDERSTANDING ALLERGY

To understand what to do to cure chronic middle ear disease, we need first to understand what allergy is all about. This chapter will introduce basic concepts that will be elaborated on in chapters that follow.

To begin, let us look at the term *inflammation*. Most people think of inflammation as it results from an infection. The tissue gets red, warm, swollen and causes pain. True infection can be caused by viruses, bacteria, parasites, fungi or other living organisms. When the mucous membrane or skin anywhere on the body is inflamed it swells with fluid and inflammatory white cells that rush to the area to protect you from assault by these organisms and other foreign intruders. Any injury such as biting your tongue, hitting your thumb with a hammer or a splinter causes the same inflammatory response to clean up damaged tissue, but this is *not* an infection.

You experience inflammation when you have a bad cold and the lining of your nose swells so much you can't even breathe through it. The same thing can happen to the lining of the tube leading to the middle ear, which is called the *Eustachian tube*. The opening to the nose is so big you can get your finger into it, and it might measure as large as eight to ten millimeters in diameter. The diameter of the opening of the Eustachian tube leading from the back of your throat to your ear is no more than two or three millimeters, so it's much easier for this tube to swell shut with just a little bit of inflammation, as explained in Chapter Five.

Allergy too is a form of inflammation that is not an infection. Allergy is the body's abnormal reaction to normal things in the environment such as dust, cats, pollen, molds, foods, and other common *allergens.* When you are allergic, your body attacks the proteins from allergens and forms antibodies. These antibodies involve a form of immunoglobulins called "Immunoglobulin E," or "IgE antibodies." They react to the proteins of an allergen and trigger your body's cells to release many different chemicals. Histamine is the major active agent in all allergy reactions; it causes the mucous membrane lining the sinuses, lungs, nose, and ears to be inflamed with swelling and increased secretions.

What is mucous membrane? Where does it come from? When we are forming as unborn babies, early in the first few weeks, the little ball of cells that will become a fetus develops an indentation and our skin turns inside itself, like forming a donut. Thus our outside skin makes the lining of all our insides — lungs, nose, and even intestines. The mucous membrane lining all our insides — from mouth and nose through the intestines — is really just skin (ectoderm) turned outside-in like a donut: the outside icing is the same as the icing on the inside of the hole. It is all skin with different names. This is important because all "skin" has the same inflammatory response to the same stimulus, no matter where it is located.

The key to understanding allergy is to remember that your mucous membrane, wherever on the body it is located, can react in only one of these two ways: First, histamine causes the mucous membrane to swell up or be congested ("inflamed"), so your nose gets stuffy. Second, histamine causes the mucous membrane to make a lot more mucus, so your nose gets runny. If the histamine attacks the mucous membrane of the nose or sinuses, we call it rhinitis or sinusitis. If it attacks the lungs, we call it asthma or allergic bronchitis. Hives and eczema are also due to excess histamine released under the skin. These diseases are simply skin hyper reactivity. All are allergic responses with different names. (And yes — some researchers have found that allergy also occurs in the mucous membrane (mucosa) lining of the intestine, as it may react to dairy or other foods like peanut products with an allergic response.)

If the histamine attacks the mucous membrane of the ear and Eustachian tube, it causes fluid behind the eardrum, or *serous otitis.* This is also an allergic disease and that is the subject of this book.

The best approach to allergies is to prevent an allergic reaction in the first place, and there are only two ways to do this. One, called "*avoidance,*" is to stay completely away from what you are allergic to, such as dust, mold, or your cat. For most people, trying to do this *is totally impractical.* The other way is to stop your body from making these extra antibodies *before* they trigger the histamines and the allergy symptoms. The only way to do this is through *immunotherapy* — the medical term for "allergy shots."

Allergy shots keep the body from making these extra antibodies. It's like turning down the volume on a radio. Immunotherapy as explained in Chapter Ten is the only way to gradually turn down your immune system so that it does not make so much "noise" in your body. Your cells no longer overreact and they stop making the antibodies that can trigger the release of more histamine. THE VISCIOUS CIRCLE IS FINALLY BROKEN.

Before one can offer immunotherapy to a patient it is essential to determine to what they are allergic. This requires some type of allergy testing which will be presented in detail later.

It should be understood that immunotherapy only affects that part of the immune system that mistakenly thinks that normal things like cats and pollen are bad. Allergy shots have no effect on that part of our immune system that we need to fight real infections. Several patients who have been on chemotherapy or even had kidney or heart transplants have successfully taken allergy shots with no ill effect on the rest of their immune system. It is even safe during pregnancy.

There are hundreds of double-blind, placebo-controlled studies in the medical literature that *prove* that allergy immunotherapy cures allergic rhinitis[3] and runny noses as well as asthma. This book is not about asthma, but it is important to note that we in the medical community understand allergy in the lung because it is responsible for as much as 90 percent of all asthma. The same process is going on in the allergic ear.

To prove how effective allergy shots are, you need look no further than the World Health Organization. Since 1998, this organization has recommended that anyone with asthma who is taking two or more medications should be considered for allergy immunotherapy. It has also been shown that immunotherapy using allergy shots will reduce the odds of developing asthma by 50 percent.[4] Sadly, doctors ignore their own "evidence-based medicine," and the makers of allergy shots don't advertise every night on the evening news, so allergy sufferers (or their anxious parents) never find out that immunotherapy works.

For some 40 percent of allergic people, the *symptoms* can be relieved temporarily with antihistamines and other medications. As stated, though, the only way to really *treat* allergy is to down-regulate the immune systems of allergic people and revert them back to a normal response either by total avoidance of the offending allergens or allergy desensitization shots — immunotherapy.

You have three choices if you have asthma or rhinitis or chronic middle ear disease; I call it…

THE 3 M'S OF TREATMENT:

1. You can be *miserable*. Just do nothing and live with your disease.
2. You can *mask* your symptoms with medication. Of course, as soon as the medicine wears off, you have to keep buying and taking more — sometimes for years.
3. You can *modify* your immune system and turn it back to normal with allergy shots.

These options are explained in detail in Chapter Nine.

How the whole allergy response is triggered is complex, so here in the first ten chapters I have simplified it for parents and patients. The scientific information, with references, is provided in more depth in *Chapter Eleven: To Your Doctor*. Take your time to read and understand it. Then you can take this whole book to your family physician or pediatrician so they can understand what you're talking about when you seek the right course of treatment for you or your child.

If you have stayed with me thus far, you already understand three simple but important concepts:

1. The whole respiratory tract is lined by mucous membrane;
2. The mucous membrane responds the same no matter where on the body it is; so,
3. The mucous membrane can react in one of two ways: normally or by becoming hyper reactive with allergy.

Now that you understand what causes asthma or sinusitis, you understand what causes middle ear disease — and you didn't even have to go to medical school!

« 2 »

ALLERGY IS HYPER REACTIVITY

Parents often ask me, "Why does my child have allergies, or asthma, or middle ear infections, or sinus disease when other children don't?" The answer is that the cells of people with allergy are *hyper reactive,* meaning they are *over reactive.* There are really only two kinds of people in the world (besides boys and girls): "NORMAL" people and ALLERGIC people. People with certain inherited genetic factors are programmed to respond to environmental allergens (such as dust, pollen, molds, pets) by making antibodies.[5] The resulting antigen (allergen) and antibody collision triggers the release of a whole different system of hyper reactive cells than seen in normal people, who do not respond to these outside factors. The *white blood cells* (used by the body to fight infections) of normal vs. allergic people behave in totally different ways. Normal people have normal white blood cells, which, if exposed to dust or pollen in the environment, do nothing. You actually are not *supposed* to react to normal things in the environment.

> Allergic people, on the other hand,
> have hyper reactive white blood cells —
> especially **mast cells** and cells called **eosinophils**.

When the cells of allergic people are exposed to dust, pollen, and other allergens in the environment, their cells overreact and release a lot of chemical substances called *mediators*. Mediators are very caustic to delicate mucous membranes, along the lines of pouring lye or Liquid-Plumr into your eyes. They create a lot of inflammation, resulting in those uncomfortable or even life-threatening reactions that bring the allergy sufferer such misery. Asthma is often called a "hyper reactive airway disease" because the airways overreact to irritation from allergens or a viral infection.

The medical fact is that the mucous membrane lining the nose, sinuses, middle ear, and lung all act the same way and all are hyper reactive in allergic people. So I like to think in the larger sense that *allergy is a hyper reactive disease of the mucous membrane* or skin — wherever that hyper reactivity is occurring in the body.

To understand the difference between normal cells and hyper reactive cells, imagine human cells as a classroom full of kindergarten children. When the teacher is in the room, the children are well behaved, sitting quietly in their seats. Then the teacher leaves the room. The children all get up and run around and there is general chaos. The teacher comes back into the room and the "normal" children settle back down, but the children with ADHD or hyperactivity don't settle down. It takes quite a while to get them back into their seats because they have just been bouncing all over the room. So it is with the hyper reactive cells of allergic children.

POTENTIATING FACTORS

Viruses or bacterial infections trigger an overreaction of the mucous membrane in allergic individuals unlike that seen in normal individuals. A huge excess of mediators and enzymes are released, and even after the infecting virus or bacteria are cleared, the mucous membrane of allergic individuals continues to produce even more enzymes and bring in even more mast cells and eosinophils to the area — so symptoms continue.

We experience the same situation in a day-care center when all of the children get a cold. The children with normal cells get over the virus in a week. The ones with allergic, hyper reactive cells overreact to the cold virus, and it is these allergic children who go on to develop middle ear infections, sinus infections, and asthma. It has been shown in both England and Finland[6, 7] that *allergic children are three to five times more likely to develop ear infections than nonallergic children.* The same happens to allergic adults. Adults with allergies learn that as soon as they get a cold, they're more likely to develop a sinus infection or have their asthma triggered, and often they need to take preventative measures such as increasing their medication or taking antibiotics.

Children in homes with cigarette smokers are twice as likely to get ear infections as children with nonsmoking parents. If those same children are allergic, they have an additional doubling of risk per pack of exposure.[8] Therefore smoking in the presence of a hyper reactive allergic child presents four times the risk for developing ear infections. I discuss additional risk factors in the last chapter, *To Your Doctor.*

Tim, age 25

Dear Dr. Hurst,

I am a 25-year-old male who has had ear problems my entire life. By the age of twelve I had already had 6 pairs of tubes put in and I have had them in and out during my entire life. I have on several occasions been tested for allergies and with the exception of when I was a young child, they always turn up negative. I've since developed my own hypothesis and I would appreciate your feedback and any information you have on scientific studies of this hypothesis.

I believe that cigarette smoke is a direct cause of Otitis Media. Why? Is it because of my experience with second-hand smoke? Both of my parents have smoked my entire life and my mother smoked during pregnancy. Of course, I had trouble my entire childhood which included hyperactivity due to medication and speech problems. The first time I can recall prolonged relief was when my parents quit smoking for approximately eight months. I was in college but living at home, and I had no sinusitis or ear problems that entire time. Then, they started smoking again. Almost immediately I was back at the doctor for the same problem. I've also noticed that my ear congestion tends to be worse the day after I go to a bar or nightclub where smoking is prevalent. I just wonder if being exposed to smoke led to the chronic problems experienced at a young age and could preventing these problems at a young age have led to better health as an adult?

Many thanks, Tim

Reply:

Hi Tim,

You are living proof of the fact that cigarette smoke is an added risk factor to those who have allergies. Smoke makes you 2-3 times more likely to have otitis than if you had only allergies. Avoiding parents who smoke is not always an option. Getting your allergies under control is therefore even more important for you if you want to stop having middle ear disease....

Dr. Hurst

Now that you know the basic terms, the answer to the question "What is allergy anyway?" can be summarized: *Allergy involves an abnormal hyper reactive response of the mucous membrane (or skin) to exposure to normal things in the environment called allergens (such as dust, pollen, and animals). This hyper reactive response of the cells of allergic people to antibodies triggers the release of histamine and other mediators because their cells have overreacted to a normal stimulus.*

And now that you understand what is meant by the word "allergy," we can go on to help you understand how what we doctors call the "allergic march" begins.

THE UNIFIED AIRWAY

Since the year 2000, both the European and American Allergy Academies have come to view the upper respiratory tract as a unified airway system. No longer should physicians behave like the nine blind men and the elephant. If you recall the poem by Rudyard Kipling, each man held a different part of the elephant. One had a leg and thought the elephant was a tree; one had the tail and thought the elephant was a snake, and so on. But unlike those blind men, we can open our eyes, stand back, and see that the nose, the lungs, the sinuses, the larynx and the middle ear are all parts of a unified respiratory system made from the same ectoderm (same part of the inside lining of the donut).

The unity of the system in response to allergies manifests itself early on as the "allergic march." Allergic infants will begin with eczema, perhaps by the age of three months. They will then gradually develop recurrent runny noses by the time they are a year old, recurrent otitis media, often with fluid (chronic middle ear fluid) by age two, and by age four, the allergic child may well begin to show signs of asthma.

These diseases may manifest themselves beginning at different ages, peak at different ages, and then resolve in a great number of individuals. Yet in others, the diseases may persist for years and years, or even crescendo as we see in asthmatics. Often asthma continues to involve more and more children as their age increases. The underlying concept is that allergy can affect different target organs at different ages, and can march along into different "diseases." All are inflammatory diseases because the cells stimulated by an allergic response release a whole host of inflammatory mediators that perpetuate mucosal inflammation. So, just as asthma is a hyper reactive disease of airway mucosa, *all* allergic disease is hyper reactive mucosal disease, regardless of the location of the mucous membrane.

One of the great unknowns in medicine is why the same person will get asthma from exposure to cats, but shrimp gives her hives. Or why when eating nuts do they get hives on 3 or 4 areas but not the whole body? All I can say is: "Thank goodness! – but we really don't know why."

When triggered by a virus, a bacterium, or histamine, any mucous membrane will react by becoming inflamed, as detailed in Chapter Five. Under those conditions, the inflamed mucous membrane swells and releases a lot of fluid that we call *mucus*. Allergy can cause the mucous membrane to swell just as effectively as a viral infection does. The poor mucous membrane of the sinuses knows only two ways to react to being irritated, whether by a virus or by histamine from allergies: swell up or make mucous.

In sinus disease, allergies can lead to stuffy noses and sinus headaches. Inflammation leads to swelling and the secretion of mucus. When this happens in the sinuses, you develop a sinus headache from the vacuum pressure. This can eventually allow a true bacterial infection to develop into a true sinus infection. Bacteria like nothing better than to set up home in a nice wet, dark basement, and your sinuses are the perfect environment. That bacterial invasion leads to a sinus infection we call sinusitis. The same vacuum pressure happens when your ears are plugged up by riding in an airplane or when you get a bad cold.

The same happens in the lungs. When you first get bronchitis or an asthma attack, the tiny air tubes leading to the lung tissue swell up and close off small portions of the lung. Increased mucus is produced, the lung fills with fluid, and it is difficult to get air into the lung. This leads to wheezing and coughing as you try to clear the fluid from the lung. If this condition persists, the obstruction leads to infection because again, the bacteria like a wet, dark, closed space to grow in. We call the infection in the lung pneumonia — but it is the result of a process identical to what we just learned happens in the sinuses.

J.S., age 29

Dear Dr. Hurst,

In the past few years, I have steadily experienced more ear/sinus problems (I am a 29-year-old female). I take various over the counter sinus medications (on a daily basis) for symptoms that include headaches, sinus pressure, stuffy nose, plugged ear (usually my right ear). The headaches and sinus pressure get much worse when the weather is bad (rain or snow).

During the week, I get up at 5:00 a.m. and usually take two sinus pills (sometimes it is necessary to take more in the afternoon). This seems to keep my symptoms at bay during the week. However, on weekends I wake up several hours later. Within an hour of getting out of bed, my right ear plugs up. It usually takes several hours to half a day for it to unplug (after taking two sinus pills). Why is this happening and what can be done about it? I'm also concerned about having to take this medication daily.

Additionally, I seem to have daily drainage...I'm constantly clearing mucus from my throat, especially after I eat a meal. I would really appreciate any advice you have for me.

Thanks, J.S.

Reply:

Dear J.S.,

When I hear the story or recurrent sinus headaches and infections I think of allergy. The fact that you can almost predict the weather because it so closely parallels your infection tells me that you are most likely allergic to molds. Check your house for water damage and get tested for allergy.

Dr. Hurst

All our medical treatments for asthmatic bronchitis are aimed to: 1) kill the bacteria with antibiotics; 2) open the passages in the lung with bronchial dilatators, or the nose with decongestants; 3) encourage cough and airway drainage; and 4) block the inflammation with steroid sprays, inhalers, and pills. Sometimes, we attempt to get air back into the lung with nebulizer treatments. If the course of treatment is not successful, the obstruction and fluid with bacteria can lead to pneumonia or even a lung abscess.

At the risk of sounding repetitive, the exact same process we observe in the sinuses and lungs also happens in an ear infection. So, infection or inflammation of the Eustachian tube initially leads to obstruction — or blockage — of the Eustachian tube, just as a cold leads to a plugged-up nose. Remember, the Eustachian tube is much smaller than the nasal passage. Just as we observed in the sinuses, if swelling from a viral cold or allergies closes the Eustachian tube, the middle ear fills with fluid. The fluid in the middle ear becomes a perfect home for bacteria, resulting in otitis media: a middle ear infection.

So now you can see that the upper respiratory tract can truly be considered a unified airway system. It is all lined by mucous membrane which responds the same to virus, bacteria or allergy no matter where it is located. The same "allergic march" that leads allergic children to develop eczema by six months, then sinusitis by 3 years, and asthma by age 6 or 7 also leads to otitis media — chronic fluid in the middle ear — when they are only two. *Obstruction leads to infection.* Sometimes it is just plain old fluid mistakenly called an "ear infection," or, as just described, it may become a true infection when bacteria invade the fluid. Either way, if the child has fluid in her ears, antibiotics will not cure the problem if the fluid is not truly infected by bacteria. Even if it *is* truly infected and antibiotics are called for in the short term, we have to find the underlying cause of the problem or it will keep recurring.

In other words, what is your child allergic to, and how do we stop the "allergic march" from taking away his right to hear properly?

First we must clear up a few misconceptions about the differences among "acute" and "chronic ear infections" and "chronic middle ear fluid."

« 3 »

HOW EARS WORK

To understand what is happening with your ears or your child's ears, we need to review the basic parts of the ear. You might remember from tenth-grade biology that the ear has three parts. What we call "the ear" is the outer ear — the part elephants can flap around. The outer ear also includes the ear canal up to the eardrum. The eardrum itself and the space that holds the delicate little bones (remember the hammer, anvil, and stirrup?) are called the *middle ear*. That is where all the disease occurs.

Beyond the middle ear are the nerve structures for hearing and balance, referred to as the *inner ear*. The hearing structure in the inner ear is shaped like a snail so it is called the *cochlea*, after a conch shell, and it is directly connected to nerve endings that control hearing and balance. Those nerves for hearing and balance come directly from the brain.

The middle ear is not a single isolated bubble, but is a rather large air- filled space the size of a half-inch-diameter marble connected to many other smaller air-filled spaces, like a sponge, called *mastoid cells*. These fill the portion of your skull that surrounds the middle ear to form the mastoid bone. A cross section of the middle ear and mastoid bone looks similar to a cross section of a lung — where all the air cells again appear to be like a sponge — but unlike a sponge they are actually connected to the main airway tube, the bronchial tube in the lung and the Eustachian tube in the ear. But draining the fluid out of the middle ear space will not drain the fluid out of the mastoid cells that are also full. That is why the recommended treatment is to put an aeration tube in the eardrum. Otherwise, the middle ear itself will just be refilled from the other smaller mastoid cells that are full of fluid. I will describe aeration tubes more fully in *Chapter Six: Treatment Options.*

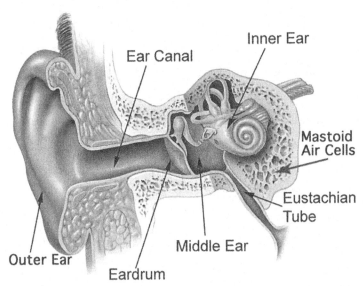

Figure 1: Diagram of ear anatomy

Where does all this fluid come from? The middle ear and all its connecting mastoid cells are lined by mucous membrane. This mucous membrane swells up and makes lots of mucus in response to any inflammation including allergies. Getting the fluid out of the middle ear and putting the tube in the eardrum for continuing airflow allows the ear function to return to normal and the hearing to return to normal.

EARS THAT GO "POP"

The middle ear space is connected to the upper part of your throat by the *Eustachian tube* (ET). The openings to the Eustachian tubes are approximately three-quarters of an inch behind your upper wisdom teeth, and the tubes are normally closed. The tubes open whenever we swallow or yawn. When you go up a long hill, you move from an area of high pressure to an area of low pressure (and vice versa going downhill). The change in air pressure creates a partial vacuum in the middle ear, which gives you the sensation that you need to "pop" them.

The same thing happens when you travel by plane. You know it is time to prepare for landing when all the little children start screaming from their earaches, and when you yourself feel an earache because of the negative pressure, or partial vacuum, in the middle ear space. You then have to try really hard to swallow or yawn to "pop your ears" as the plane lands so as to let air come up the Eustachian tubes.

If we are unable to get air up the tube, the oxygen in the middle ear and mastoid cells is absorbed and a vacuum is created. This causes increased discomfort, and the vacuum will actually suck fluid from the lining of the middle ear into the cavity itself. The ear will fill with thin, clear fluid that is sterile (though later on this fluid can be inoculated by bacteria, which results in infection). Doctors call this fluid an "effusion."

Doctors are always jumping to "the cure." But first we need to answer the question "Why is this happening?" The basic problem responsible for ear disease is that something makes it hard for the Eustachian tube to open easily. There are a number of reasons why an ear may not be working correctly and eventually becomes "infected" or has fluid. Usually a viral cold in an infant or allergy as children get bigger is the cause of swelling of the ET so it cannot open. This is discussed in detail in Chapter Eleven under *Mechanisms responsible for Otitis Media with Effusion*. The success of various treatment options depends on your doctor making the correct diagnosis — not of the problem, but the *cause* of the problem. The most obvious and most common cause for our ears not to work is a true upper respiratory tract infection – a "cold." *But it persists and fails to clear if you have allergies.*

« 4 »

EAR INFECTIONS
ACUTE OR CHRONIC?

What's in a name? The term "ear infection" is a broad and sometimes imprecise label. Actually, acute and chronic ear infections are two separate diseases. Doctors often simplistically and incorrectly put both in the same basket and call them "ear infections." This is like a child calling appendicitis a "stomach ache." Most ear infections come on suddenly with pain. Although acute infections are not the focus of this book, I think it is important to understand the basics about recurrent acute infections.

Often your doctor will say that your child has an ear infection, meaning a sudden process where your child wakes up with pain; the eardrum looks red or is even bulging with pus. The child is very uncomfortable, crying at night, and runs a fever. This is considered an *acute ear infection.* "Acute" refers to the first day or two of sudden discomfort. They are of short duration. Most of these recurrent acute ear infections will resolve spontaneously, that is, without medical intervention, most of the time.

An acute infection of the middle ear, called *acute otitis media,* is very common in infants. Thirty-five percent of preschool-age children experience an ear infection. Viruses are the cause of half of these, so antibiotics will do no good half of the time. Eighty-three percent will resolve in three days with no treatment. There is realistic concern about the frequent use of antibiotics creating resistant strains of bacteria. This has put pressure on physicians to minimize the use of antibiotics, so current guidelines[2] advise that they be withheld for the first 24 hours of an acute otitis media. Only if continual pain or fever persists, unassociated with a chest cold, for more than two days should antibiotics be prescribed. Though it is rare for an acute infection to go on to significant complications, such as mastoiditis or meningitis, a physician should see a child who continues to run a fever and has discomfort for more than 48 hours.

Most allergic children initially present with infection.

Child, 13 months

Dear Dr. Hurst,

My daughter is 13 months old and has suffered from OME since the age of 4 months. She has had an average of 2 ear infections per month. My pediatrician has spoken to me about tubes on several occasions, but now she does not respond to the same medication twice in a row. For example, she was on Zithromax for 5 days and then we waited 5 days and started it again as a preventive. During the 2nd administration of it she developed a severe infection in the right ear. She is now finishing up the Vantin and seems to be clear. The pediatrician has recommended an ENT (who is not an allergist) to do the surgery and I am having trouble finding an ENT allergist in my area. I am skeptical of tubes because I do not feel it is a solution to the problem, only to the symptom. Is 13 months young to have tubes placed?

Thanks again and Happy New Year.

Barbara, Pompano Beach, FL

Reply:

There are basically 2 types of ear infections: Your daughter shows the first type—that is recurrent infections, one right after another, which usually clear in 1-2 weeks. These are the children who are most easily cured by tympanostomy or aeration (a hole in the eardrum) tubes. If your daughter not only has recurrent infections, but also does not clear easily, then she may ALSO have allergies.

Dr. Hurst

Chronic ear infection describes one of two possible scenarios: The term may refer to the situation wherein a patient experiences multiple acute infections. These happen one after another so the ear inflammation presents as "chronically recurrent" disease. Or sometimes "chronic ear infection" refers to a persistent, acute ear infection that has not resolved after four to eight weeks and thus has become "chronic" or long-lasting.

Children in the first instance with chronic ear infections have a series of acute infections that seem to improve; yet in one to four weeks they get a repeat infection. If this happens with enough frequency — typically when a child has had five or six *recurrent-acute* infections within a year — most ear doctors would suggest placing *middle ear tubes*, the technical term being *tympanostomy tubes*. The tubes, placed in the eardrums, are a simple way to bypass the Eustachian tube obstruction and provide a route for air to come in from the outside. This prevents about 80 percent of the recurring ear infections.

The second category involves middle ear fluid that persists. Following an acute infection about 20 percent of children will retain the fluid in their ears for two or three months. Also, there is a small group of patients who present with fluid in their ears which seems to have occurred without ever having had an infection. These children or adults never had an earache. They just suddenly are not hearing well and are found to have fluid behind their eardrums. This is also called a "chronic middle ear infection" though there may actually be no bacteria in the middle ear. That is, the fluid is usually sterile, but the persistence of that fluid for two or three months is called a chronic "infection." In this instance, using the word infection leads to confusion because the ear is not technically infected at all. But it *is* INFLAMED. *Almost all of these patients have been proven to have allergy as the cause for this inflammation.*

Of the 17 percent of children who have chronic fluid in the ear following an acute infection that did not clear, only 26 percent will resolve within six months, meaning the fluid clears on its own with no medical intervention. (Figure 2) The median duration of un-

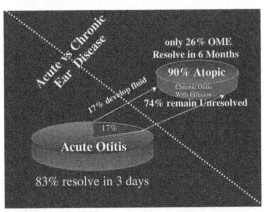

Figure 2: Acute Otitis Media vs. Otitis Media with Effusion

treated otitis media with effusion is reported to be a staggering 6.1 to 7.8 years. This means that nearly three-fourths of affected children will maintain fluid in their ears for more than a year.[9] *Therefore, of the four million children in the United States (alone) who develop chronic fluid in their ears — three million will not clear spontaneously and will continue to suffer for years with persistent fluid and its accompanying hearing loss.*

My point is: *all this is preventable.*

It astonishes me that my fellow doctors can tell the parents of these children, "Oh, don't worry about a little fluid in the ear. It won't bother them." Your own experience should tell you that having fluid in your ears is annoying and even painful. Most of us have gone swimming and come out with a little water left in our ears. We do this great rain dance, jumping up and down to shake the water out of our ears because it drives us crazy. That awfully annoying sensation and hearing loss are intolerable to an adult. How can we allow three million children to go a year (or more) with fluid in their ears before removing it? I don't understand it. *As mentioned earlier, chronic fluid in the ear can lead to hearing loss, delayed speech, and accompanying learning disabilities, all of which are avoidable or reversible.*

OK, let's think about the way children with additional learning and behavior disabilities are further handicapped by poor hearing. In this regard, 2 + 2 = 8. That is, one problem is not just *added* to another problem, but *compounds* the situation with many more difficulties. The fluid causes as much hearing loss as having a good set of ear plugs in your ears. Children with learning or behavior problems have trouble enough processing what they would hear normally. It is even more important that these kids with special needs be given every opportunity to maximize their potential. That is impossible if they don't hear correctly. I recently had a 4-year-old boy with ADHD who'd had effusion for the previous two years — since his second set of tubes fell out. His speech was almost unintelligible, almost as bad as his 1-1/2-year-old brother. Within 4 months on sublingual drops for his allergies, and avoiding eggs, his speech was near normal and his nasal congestion was gone. I've seen many two- year-olds who were not talking at all, and as soon as their tubes were placed and the fluid removed, their speech normalized within a month!

It is important to understand that a "chronic middle ear infection" simply:

a) may not be an infection at all, and actually

b) refers to either frequently recurring, acute *true* infections, or

c) a persistent middle ear infection that simply hasn't cleared and presents as a middle ear with persistent fluid in it.

The latter cases are the most difficult for physicians to deal with, and most vexing for parents. These are the cases I have spent the last twenty-five years of my life trying to understand. *Chronic fluid in the ear is most difficult for physicians to treat if they refuse to recognize the underlying allergy that leads to this disease.*

Child, 18 months

My 18 months girl has been having an ear infection almost every month since she was 6 months old. I have taken her to her doctor, who's a Swedish consultant (pediatric), and each time he would prescribe an antibiotic. I've asked him if that might have been related to some kind of an allergy (because she has a lot of food allergies and her infections are accompanied with skin rashes or eczema), and he almost laughed at me, saying that it's bacteria that cause the infection and it's not related to allergy! I've decided to do my own research and I found your site on the Internet. We stopped her milk and cheese and both the eczema and ear fluid cleared. She has not been sick for 6 months.

E. Al-Bedah, Kuwait

« 5 »

INFLAMMATION
INFECTION OR ALLERGY?

Understanding allergy requires an understanding of the basic fact that the entire upper airway – the nose, sinuses, bronchial tubes, and middle ear space – are all lined with mucous membrane. Your mucous membrane can only respond to an insult from bacteria, a virus, foreign body or an allergic reaction by *inflammation*. The chemicals released bring in white cells, increase the local blood flow (causing redness), increase fluid (causing more swelling), and increase mucus production. In the lung we call this reaction asthma; in the nose we call it rhinitis or sinusitis; in the eye we call it conjunctivitis; *and in the ear it leads to middle ear fluid that we call otitis media.*

The "*itis*" on the end of a word, as in sinusitis, rhinitis, conjunctivitis, or otitis, *implies infection, but really means inflammation.* This is an important technical distinction because if the inflammation is truly infection from bacteria, antibiotics will work. However, if the "itis"/inflammation is not bacterial but rather from a foreign body (such as sand in your eye or a splinter in your finger), antibiotics obviously will not work.

In the case of a bacterial invasion, antibodies bring in white cells to kill the bacteria. This produces dead white cells that we call pus. When inflammation is caused by antibodies responding in an allergic reaction, the antibodies recruit different kinds of white cells that release more chemical mediators, causing even more *inflammation*. This produces more swelling, more mucus, and fluid production in the area, causing you to sneeze and have a runny nose.

A foreign body like sand in your eye can cause *inflammation* of the lining of the eye - conjunctivitis. Actually the conjunctiva is just a thin layer, one cell thick, of mucous membrane covering the whites of your eyes. When the conjunctiva is irritated, it swells. The eye appears to turn red and produces a lot of tearing.

The same thing happens in the lining of the nose if a foreign body tickles the mucous membrane. You sneeze because of the watery mucus, irritation, and swelling, or you cough and constantly clear your throat because of the mucous dripping down the back of your throat from your sinuses. The same initial reaction to a foreign body in the lung causes coughing, watery discharge, and a great deal of discomfort. *An allergen, be it in the form of pollen, dog dander, dust, or mold, is a foreign body that can irritate the lining of the eye, nose, lung, and middle ear in an identical manner.* This irritation again causes *inflammation*.

> You will understand why taking antibiotics for otitis media caused by allergies will do no good whatsoever if you remember that
> - *antibiotics* are used for *bacterial infection* and
> - *antihistamines* are used (but don't always work well) for *allergy*.

It is interesting that twenty-five years ago, all the allergy literature said allergy had absolutely nothing to do with asthma, because researchers couldn't find any evidence in the lung of allergy chemicals or mediators. Then suddenly twenty years ago, allergists made a 180-degree turnaround, and now everyone agrees that as much as 90 percent of asthma is allergy related. That is because we can now identify various chemical mediators that are classic markers of allergy. These markers are cellular fingerprints. They are as specific as DNA. Each is distinct for an individual cell that is found only in specific circumstances. Those same cellular markers for allergy have been found in the noses and sinuses of patients with allergic rhinitis.

You might have wondered why allergic people react to allergens at some times, but don't react every time they are exposed to a particular allergen. I like to compare the mucous membrane to a mousetrap. A mousetrap sometimes has a stiff spring and isn't triggered even by an aggressive mouse, which gets away with the cheese. At other times the mousetrap has a hair trigger and snaps at the slightest jiggling, sometimes before you can get it down on the floor. Once it does snap, the reaction in either situation is the same: BANG! Sometimes allergic people are triggered by a tiny bit of allergen, and sometimes it takes a whole lot before they are triggered. But once the mucous membrane is triggered, the reaction again is the same, whether it is in the lung, nose, eye, sinus, or middle ear. There will be a release of chemicals to bring in more cells, and more blood flow, and a release of fluid and mucus that will cause swelling.

BUT WHAT ABOUT THE MIDDLE EAR?

As much as it had been theorized that allergy had some connection to middle ear disease, there had never been proof of a chemical marker of allergic inflammatory activity in the middle ear itself — so I set out to find one.

My thinking twenty years ago was that allergy must be causing some cases of chronic middle ear disease, but we hadn't been able to identify any of the mediators. *My research, and research done by others, demonstrated that exactly the same cells and exactly the same chemical mediators found in the lung and sinuses in allergic disease are also found in the middle ear.*

Unfortunately, some medical practices have not kept pace with the research. Ear doctors are about fifteen years behind lung doctors, and it was only in 2004 that an official acknowledgement came from the Academy of Otolaryngology (ear doctors), the Academy of General Family Practice, and the Academy of Pediatrics: "The middle ear is capable of an allergic response."[2] This statement is the first official recognition that the mucous membrane in the middle ear behaves like all the rest of the mucous membrane in the lungs and sinuses, and that the middle ear can indeed participate in an allergic reaction. This statement is as momentous as the declaration that the world is round or that Earth is not the center of the solar system! (It might be noted that the above declaration by the three academies cited three of my studies[1, 10, 11] as references upon which their statement was based.)

So, what does this mean for patients? It means that the lining of the middle ear and Eustachian tube is identical to the lining of the sinuses and the lung. If your child is allergic, when he is exposed to allergens such as dust, pollen, or cats, and his body makes antibodies to those allergens, those antibodies can cause the lining of the middle ear to release histamine and other chemicals that result in swelling and/or mucus production in the middle ear itself — just as these would in the sinuses or lungs.

> **There is one great difference between the middle ear and the sinuses and lungs:**
> *there is no way for the fluid to get out of the middle ear!*

If you have extra fluid in your sinuses and your nose, you blow it out. If you have extra fluid in your lungs, you cough it out. But if there is extra fluid in your middle ear, it can't get out, and so you develop "chronic infection" or "effusion" with fluid and hearing loss. If you or your child is in this category, and you understand this truth with just the basic terminology I have reviewed thus far, you are ahead of many physicians. And if your child's doctor cannot understand it, even after reading the chapter at the end of this book explaining in detail the science behind what I have just said, it's time to find a new doctor.

Let's look more closely at middle ear infection. As stated previously, the term "chronic" is used to describe two situations: either the patient has repeated infections and/or a single acute infection hasn't cleared, meaning that all the fluid hasn't cleared. That fluid no longer has bacteria in it (i.e., the fluid is sterile). The ear with fluid in it for more than two months is considered to have a "chronic middle ear disease infection," when in actuality it is not infected at all; it is just chronic in terms of time.

This is important for two reasons:
- This fluid **leads to hearing loss**, and
- The fluid is **not going to go away by itself**; it must be removed.

The only way to remove fluid from the middle ear is to make a small hole in the eardrum to suction that fluid out and possibly put in a tube.

I tell my patients that putting in the aeration tube buys us about a year of time, because usually the tube stays in for about a year or a year and a half. That gives us ample time to determine whether the child has allergies, and if so, to get the allergies under control. Then, when the tube comes out, the fluid won't recur.

Child, age 11

Dear Dr. Hurst:

I am just writing to give you a summary of our past experience with our 11-year-old son. As a baby he had experienced several bouts of infection and fluid in the middle ear. The specialist finally inserted tubes after a tonsil and adenoidectomy at 2 years old. Since then he has had 10 insertions of tubes, sometimes in one ear and sometimes in both. He does well while the tubes are in place but they do tend to come out on their own and he is OK for a while, but then the hearing decreases and symptoms show that he is again due for another recheck. We make visits to the audiologists to keep a check on the amount of hearing loss and usually it is no more then 35% in one ear and that is usually the worst. The doctor's last comment when I asked how much longer we would keep inserting these tubes was "until he stops needing them." No one has ever mentioned allergies to us as being the cause, and the specialist thought he would have outgrown the need for tubes before this. Any comments you have would be appreciated.

PEI (Prince Edward Island)
Canada

Reply:

DEAR PEI:

Your child has allergies and needs a full evaluation for inhalants and food allergy before he has 11 sets of tubes!!

As for multiple tube insertions. There can be some scarring, but the bigger danger—especially with the "permanent tubes," or large bore tubes/grommets, is that they have a 30% or greater chance of permanent perforation if left after 6 months. Better the smaller tubes more frequently—they will buy you a year to find his ALLERGIES.

Your comment that he has "ONLY 35% HEARING LOSS" is most frightening. We know that hearing loss in one ear for 3 months leads to speech and language delay. Fortunately your son is brighter than the average and is getting by in the system—but still not learning all that he is capable of learning. He will need another—and hopefully last—set of tubes to buy time to evaluate and treat his allergies.

Good luck.

Dr. Hurst

« 6 »

TREATMENT OPTIONS

We have learned that the term "ear infection" covers a range of situations from acute (sudden and painful) recurring episodes of infection to persistent fluid in the ear that may last for months and months. There are a variety of treatments offered and patients and/or their parents need to know when it is appropriate to consider antibiotics, ear tubes, tonsillectomy, osteopathic or chiropractic manipulation, antihistamines, corticosteroids, or even middle ear surgery. Let's evaluate each option.

ACUTE INFECTIONS

A historical perspective: When your infant awakens in the middle of the night screaming, holding her ear and running a fever, and the doctor finds her eardrum is bright red or bulging with pus, your child is suffering from an acute ear infection. Before the age of antibiotics, and even up until the 1970s, the standard of care was to hold the child down on the exam table and lance the eardrum to let the pus out, just like lancing a boil. The pain would cease, the ear would drain for a day or two, and the ear infection would resolve. Barbaric but effective.

Child, age 4½

Dear Dr. Hurst:

I have a four-and-a-half-month-old daughter who has had a chronic ear infection since practically birth. She has had a total of five different antibiotics and is currently taking Vantin. My pediatrician stated that if that doesn't work, he wants to consider putting tubes in. He feels that she is pretty young and would prefer to wait until she is a year old, but since the ears are not clearing, he feels he does not have a choice. She was born only two weeks premature (8 lbs. at birth) but with respiratory distress syndrome, and spent 11 days in the NICU, five of them on a respirator. She received intravenous antibiotics during that time.

My questions are: Did her time in the NICU cause or contribute to her ear problems? Is she really too young for tubes? (I sincerely hope not... I would like her to feel better and her screaming is making me crazy.) Is it possible that she has a food allergy? She got breast milk for approximately three weeks and then Nutramigen formula and is now on Lacto-Free formula.

Sincerely, B.J.

Reply:

Dear B.J.

It is doubtful the NICU had any effect—and certainly not her prematurity. Infants with this much ear disease usually are allergic to the milk, and your peds is right to try the Nutramigen. Did that help? If not, then probably tubes by age 7-10 mos. is reasonable.

Dr. Hurst

In the mid-1970s, several studies indicated that Amoxicillin treatment for ten days was the best antibiotic of choice, and that has remained the standard of care for over thirty years. Now, because of increasing antibiotic resistance, the immediate use of antibiotics is being questioned for treatment of an acute infection, especially since we now know that 83 percent of these ear infections will resolve with no medical treatment.

In Europe the standard of care is to wait at least 24 to 48 hours before antibiotics are prescribed, unless pain and fever persist. In the United States there is a trend to adopt the same standard of watchful waiting for a day or two while withholding antibiotics, unless there is continued fever and pain, which can indicate a more serious condition. Occasionally, a child is put on antibiotics for one or more months in order to *prevent* recurrent infection. This is called "prophylaxis." It works in fewer than 30 percent of cases, and is not supported by current guidelines. Furthermore, inappropriate use of antibiotics leads to the development of antibiotic-resistant bacteria.

TUBES

The function of tubes is to simply bypass the Eustachian tube (blocked by inflammation of infection or allergy). They provide another way to get air into the middle ear. Aeration tubes are ideal for children with recurrent acute otitis media. Studies have shown that children who have had aeration tubes have had no permanent scarring and their hearing is no different than that of children who never had to have tubes.

In a study done in Italy in the early 1970s, one group of children with recurrent acute otitis received tubes and another group did not. The study was stopped after the first fifty children. *There was such a huge beneficial effect from the tubes, it was deemed unethical to withhold the placement of tubes from the control group of children. More than 80 percent of those children with tubes stopped having infections. Those without the tubes continued to suffer until they, too, received the tubes.*

Child, 2½ years

Dear Dr. Hurst:

I have a 2-1/2-year-old daughter, and she is constantly telling me her ears hurt. At one point when she was about 16 months old, she had so many ear infections that at 19 months they inserted the tubes in both ears and she was a totally different kid. The whining stopped, she talked better. She even ate better.

Sometimes children with tubes will continue to experience true ear infections, often in association with a cold or sinusitis. With the tubes in place the pus can drain, so there is no pressure and no pain associated with the infection. This "infection" may then resolve with antibiotic ear drops.

Occasionally, children with tubes experience recurrent drainage seemingly spontaneously. This is frequently blamed on swimming or getting water in the ears in the shower, but excellent studies have shown that to be a myth. There is the same frequency of drainage among children who are very careful and swim with

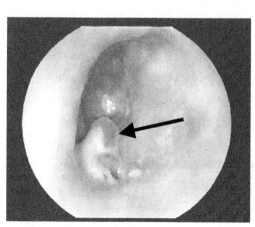

Figure 3: Draining Tube

ear plugs as there is among those who do not protect their ears from water. So if getting water in the ear and down the tube is not the reason the tube will drain, what is the reason? Think about it – perhaps this is because the percentage of swimmers with allergies is the same as the percentage among non-swimmers.

My experience, and that of others, has been that half of infants or toddlers who have recurrent acute otitis episodes every few weeks or those whose tubes continue to have intermittent drainage often have food allergies.[12] When we identify the offending food and remove it from the diet, the drainage stops.

Jacob, 14 months

I had known Jacob almost since he had been born, as he was the son of a physician friend of mine. This boy had had recurrent acute infections every four to six weeks since age 6 months. He also had colic beginning at age 3 months. He also had bright red face cheeks because of his eczema. In between his ear infections his fluid seemed not to clear. They brought him in at age 14 months.

It's very difficult to take a history from an infant. Sitting in his stroller Jacob told me all I needed to know. Red-faced and screaming he threw his baby bottle across the room. That told us! He simply didn't like the milk! I suggested we stop his dairy products and switched him to soy milk. The colic stopped. The ears cleared. His facial eczema disappeared.

He has since graduated high school with no further ear problems.

To summarize before we move on: The child with recurrent acute infections should be treated with antibiotics and/or tympanostomy tubes, according to the advice of your pediatrician, and after consultation with an ENT surgeon. Other reasons for the ears to fail to work properly include adenoid obstruction and allergies which will be considered next.

CHRONIC MIDDLE EAR DISEASE

How can we help these children with persistent fluid in the middle ear — chronic otitis that does not clear spontaneously?

A classic example of chronic middle ear disease is the child who at age 7 or 8 fails his school hearing test and is found to have fluid behind his eardrum. Yet when questioned, the parents say he/she has never had an ear infection. Often that child had been doing poorly in school to the point of being held back a year or labeled as having Attention Deficit Disorder. *The child could not hear.* So how could he/she follow instructions or complete assignments correctly?

(Little boys who can't hear entertain themselves. They become disruptive and often become labeled falsely as ADHD. Little girls who don't hear just sit quietly. They are just "so good!" – but fail to learn.)

MEDICAL MANAGEMENT

Initially decongestants containing pseudoephedrine, the active ingredient in Sudafed, may work, especially if the fluid resulted from a cold where the whole head was congested and the Eustachian tube obstructed. Sometimes at the beginning of a severe allergy season, such as when grass pollinates in the spring or ragweed in the summer, head congestion will lead to middle ear congestion. In rare cases where the fluid is caught early, an antihistamine will be of benefit.

Studies that purport to prove that antihistamines or corticosteroids are of no value did not select patients with allergy. Rather, they took all patients with otitis media. That is like saying that antibiotics don't work for pneumonia and not eliminating patients who had viral infections. Treatment studies must be read with a critical eye. Most of these studies are sponsored by drug companies trying to prove that their competition is ineffective. Good studies must be designed to eliminate this type of flawed logic, which produces flawed conclusions.

TUBES FOR CHRONIC DISEASE

If the fluid is causing hearing loss — which will certainly interfere with attention at school or one's ability to work as an adult —*the physician's first obligation to the patient is to restore normal hearing.* That is best done by putting aeration tubes in the ears.

Tubes are appropriate for children who have chronic fluid in their ears because while allowing the fluid to drain, they also allow air to get into the middle ear and the whole set of connected mastoid cells.

To place the tubes in the ear, the surgeon makes a small three-millimeter hole in the eardrum and the fluid is suctioned out. Then a tiny plastic tube is placed in the hole. This can actually be done under local anesthesia in most people over 12 or 14 years old. (Small children of course require general anesthesia.) These tubes look like a thread bobbin for a sewing machine, and measure four millimeters across with a two-millimeter opening. (In fact, in England these are called "ear bobbins.") These tubes are designed to be "shed" spontaneously by the body after a year or so. Since the hole will close in a few hours, a tube is placed in the hole to allow the whole middle ear, including those small mastoid air cells connected to it, to drain and dry. The advantage of the tube is that it not only allows the fluid to be suctioned out, but hearing is restored immediately.

Child, age 5

Subject: Your theory on Allergy as cause of OME with effusion.

Dr. Hurst,

My five-year-old daughter has been diagnosed with OM with effusion in both ears. A hearing test today confirmed significant hearing loss in both ears. Otherwise she is healthy and fine. However, this diagnosis was discovered after I consulted an ENT doctor because of a persistent nasal congestion that several doses of antibiotics (prescribed by a pediatrician) would not clear up. He gave her a nasal spray that he said only works for allergies. So I am pretty sure that she has allergies. (There is also a history of allergies on her father's side.) Anyway, the ENT and audiologist recommend tubes. I am really not happy about that and have been searching the Internet for alternative treatment, but besides your page, everyone recommends tubes more or less. I really don't know what to do. She has just started kindergarten and I don't want her to be disadvantaged because of her hearing. However, I am really concerned about the traumatic experience of surgery. I am very open to suggestions at this point. Maybe you can find the time to answer me. I would really appreciate it. Thanks a lot.

Mrs. I.G., Middletown

Reply:

It is essential to return your daughter's hearing to normal. Follow the advice and trust your ENT surgeon. You need to put in the tubes so as to 1) restore normal hearing and 2) remove the fluid, which contains very caustic enzymes and chemicals which perpetuate the inflammation. That will buy you a year to diagnose what her allergies are and get them treated.

Good Luck,
Dr. Hurst

Additionally, there are so-called "permanent tubes" designed *not* to be shed. These are either made of stainless steel or a longer, wider (12mm x 4mm vs. the standard tube of 4mm x 2mm) plastic tube with a wide flange. They do indeed stay in longer, but have a complication of leaving a permanent eardrum perforation 30 percent or more of the time when they do get pushed out. This compares to a perforation rate of only about 1 percent for standard tubes.

One of the great myths is that children with recurrent ear infections have "small Eustachian tubes." Anatomic studies done almost thirty years ago proved that the entire length of the Eustachian tube is no different in children with recurrent ear infections than it is in normal children.[13]

Another myth is that there is a difference in the Eustachian tubes of children with recurrent infections as compared with those who do not get infections. This has also been proven false.[14]

As a physician I have an obligation to strongly advise the use of tubes in the proper circumstances – but do not get me wrong. As an advocate for tubes I warn my patients that they are only by-passing the problem. I tell my patients that once the tube is in, it will stay for at least a year or more, which gives us time to find the underlying cause. Again, the issue is not just *what* treatment is indicated for the fluid, but *why* the individual is in this predicament in the first place. During the year the tube is in, we have adequate time to do an appropriate diagnostic evaluation to look for causes of the Eustachian tube obstruction. This brings us to tonsils, adenoids, and allergies.

TONSILS, ADENOIDS, AND ALLERGIES

What about the tonsils? You may have noticed I have not said anything about the tonsils causing nasal or Eustachian tube obstruction. *Tonsils*, easily seen in the mirror, are two pieces of tissue, each about the size of the end of your thumb. Tonsils and adenoids are both made of lymph-node-like tissue and reside in the back of the mouth. (Lymph nodes filter infections.) They may have little pockets in them and will swell up with streptococcus infections. Among children 2 to 4 years old, the tonsils get quite large, and then shrink again until about age 7 to 8, when they enlarge again for another year or so. There is no prize for size. ENT surgeons usually do not advise removing tonsils unless the patient has had nine tonsil infections, either three infections per year for three years, or four one year and five the next. Another indication to remove tonsils in infants and toddlers is if they are causing airway obstruction and interfering with sleep. This is something that should be discussed with your pediatrician and ENT surgeon.

Many studies have shown that tonsils have nothing to do with recurrent acute ear infections, and tonsils certainly have nothing to do with chronic middle ear fluid. *Simply put, tonsils DO NOT— and CANNOT—cause Eustachian tube obstruction or middle ear disease.*

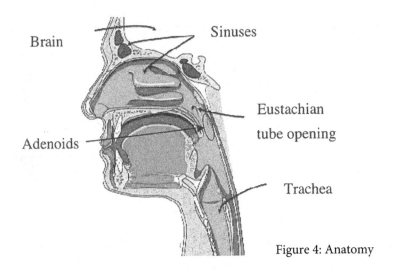

Brain

Sinuses

Eustachian
tube opening

Adenoids

Trachea

Figure 4: Anatomy

The *adenoid* pad of lymphoid tissue is high in the middle of the back wall of your mouth, just above your soft palate and behind your nose. If it is really enlarged, the adenoids may then protrude below the soft palate where they can be easily seen when your doctor uses a tongue depressor and has the child say "Aahh."

Young children who come to their doctors with *nasal obstruction* should be evaluated for enlarged adenoids. Nasal obstruction in children can only be caused by either (or both) of two things: 1) the back of the nose is obstructed by the adenoid tissue, and/or 2) the child has allergies.

A better way to check the adenoids may be to take a side view X-ray of the head and neck. That will show if the adenoids are obstructing the airway.

If the adenoids are large enough, they may overgrow and obstruct the opening of

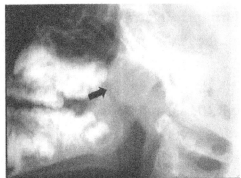

Figure 5: Adenoids on X-ray. Arrow points to adenoid pad, dark narrow streak is airway.

the Eustachian tubes. In this situation, adenoids may be a definite cause of recurrent ear infections and fluid in the ear. Of course, some children will present with both nasal obstruction from adenoids and recurrent tonsillitis, so it is appropriate to remove both tonsils and adenoids. These children deserve to be considered for placement of aeration tubes as well as removal of their adenoids. Appropriate medical treatment must be tailored to the individual situation. That is where consultation with your ear, nose, and throat surgeon is of benefit. *No matter which specialist you consult, if the answer does not make sense to you, **get a second opinion**. This is your child and you need to feel comfortable in knowing that you are doing the right thing for him or her.*

It is certainly the standard of care to remove the adenoids in children who need a second set of tubes. If the child has obvious nasal obstruction, this surgery may be appropriate even when the first set is put in. The thinking behind this is that the adenoids themselves, by their location, can block the opening of the Eustachian tube and by that alone cause chronic OME. It is certainly recognized by all pediatricians and ENT surgeons that chronic otitis media is the result of something obstructing the Eustachian tube. What they fail to do is think about what else might be causing the obstruction if it is not the adenoids. That is, they never consider allergies in these cases.

ALLERGIES

Allergies can cause the adenoids not only to swell, but also to actually regrow. Adenoids disappear at puberty, so children over 12 or 14 normally do not have any adenoid tissue left to explain their Eustachian tube obstruction. If they do still have adenoids, they definitely have allergies. I actually removed adenoids for a third time in a 17-year-old who had not been treated for his allergies. *Any child who*

*needs their adenoids removed more than once absolutely has allergies
until proven otherwise.*

GASTRO-ESOPHAGEAL REFLUX (GERD)

Gastro-esophageal reflux is another contributing factor to some
middle ear inflammation. When I was a resident forty years ago, it
was shown that infants lying on their backs and taking a bottle would
often get milk — and stomach acid from reflux or vomiting — up
into their Eustachian tubes and into their middle ears. Many children experience this reflux, and perhaps 10 percent with chronic ear
disease have been shown to have it.[15] Then, of course, there is the
question of those many children with reflux who have NO otitis
episodes. What makes them different from the otitis group? Perhaps
they have no allergies. No one has looked at how having no allergies
may *protect* those with reflux from getting ear infections.

CLEFT PALATE

There is a special group of children born with the congenital abnormality of a cleft of the soft palate and sometimes, unfortunately, a
cleft lip. They always get chronic effusions. Here's why: The muscle
that opens the Eustachian tube comes from the middle ear, travels
down along the tube itself, and swings across the mouth. It crosses
the palate and forms a sling — attaching to the same muscle coming
from the other side. This sling is in fact your soft palate. The muscles
pull against each other to open the Eustachian tube. Like grabbing
your two hands together and pulling, if you break your grip, you
cannot pull. So in the case of a cleft palate, the muscles have nothing
to pull against and so the Eustachian tubes never open. These children need aeration tubes as infants, but after the palate has been
repaired, they rarely need tubes again. There are, however, some
children who despite surgical closure of their cleft continue to have

effusion. I have had several who do not clear until, again, their allergies are controlled. Then they also no longer need tubes.

Adult, age 48

I am a 48 year-old female who has suffered from repeated ear infections all my life. I have been on numerous antibiotics that will briefly clear my ears. At present, I have vertigo from fluid in my ears. I accessed your site, and I am in total agreement with you on allergies. I am diagnosed with allergies. I had to do this because of nearly fatal episodes with asthma over the years. I have had years of sneezing until I could barely think. Doctors would medicate me with antihistamines until I would be nearly incoherent. When I got the asthma and nasal and sinus problems seemingly under control, the stuff seemed to move to my ears with a vengeance. I am tired of putting up with this. I found one doctor that listened to me. The entire right side of my head was sore and I had immense pressure from fluid in my right ear. He put a tube in my ear, which brought me almost immediate relief from pressure. And, he prescribed an antihistamine.

An antihistamine a day was working for me. Usually, 30 of them would get me through the worst of the allergy season. They did not make my kidneys hurt or give me any other miserable side effects. I hope this helps someone else. I went through years of having vertigo and being miserable. I would not wish it on anyone.

Thank you for your time.

Fairview, TN

VERTIGO

The topic of vertigo is complex and not the subject for in-depth review in this book, yet it has been reported[16] that as many as half of patients with vertigo have food allergies. True vertigo is defined as a sensation or hallucination of spinning. Occasionally a patient will report having vertigo or feeling dizzy when they have fluid in their ears. Uneven pressure on one side with fluid against the inner ear can trigger a sensation of imbalance. Certainly we have seen toddlers actually toddle when one side is infected. Adults can report this symptom, too, but remember: allergy is a diagnosis of exclusion, and persistent vertigo needs to be evaluated for other significant problems. Not everything is caused by allergy.

An important word of caution: Very rarely, an adult may present with fluid behind only one eardrum. The underlying ET obstruction may be the result of a rare tumor growing high in the back of the nose or throat. In other cases, the Eustachian tube may be scarred closed by radiation therapy to a tumor in the back of the nose or base of the brain. These are rare events, but every ENT surgeon thinks of these causes. That is why a thorough examination by a specialist is necessary. Having done that exam and found no radiation scarring, tumor, or adenoids, one must evaluate for allergies. That is the only other cause of Eustachian tube obstruction.

Now it is time to answer the five critical questions parents need to ask their child's doctor:

- **Why does the fluid form?**
- **Why don't the ears clear?**
- **Why do the tubes drain?**
- **Why don't the ears stay healthy?**
- **Why does this recur in my child when other children get better and *stay* better?**

« 7 »

ALLERGY TESTING

WHY, HOW AND WHAT KIND
— PRICK, INTRADERMAL AND RAST —

The answer to the questions raised in the previous chapter can be summed up in one word — *allergies*. If you think you or your child falls into this category, it is vital that you find the right kind of specialist to do the right kind of allergy testing so you can get to the bottom of why the fluid is forming, why it does not clear, why, if there are already tubes in the ears, they continue to drain, and why your ears or your child's ears do not get healthy and stay healthy like "normal" people's ears do.

If you even have to *ask* these questions, you absolutely need to know how to choose the right kind of allergy test and the right specialist to do the testing, and why it must be an ENT allergist trained by the American Academy of Otolaryngic Allergy or the Pan American Allergy Society.

I'll try to explain the differences between and the benefits of each type of testing. Once you understand which is the most sensitive and accurate type of test, you will understand how to choose the type of specialist you want to do your testing.

I need to pause a moment to explain an academic word game. Technically "atopic" means "reactive." An atopic patient has a positive test of some type. The term "allergy" refers to a reaction that causes symptoms. I test positive for dog, but dogs never bother me. Therefore I am atopic but not allergic to dogs. So a patient with five positive tests is atopic, yet we do not know for certain which allergen is responsible for her sneezing and which for her itchy eyes. So how can one test to see if a patient is allergic? In this book I am going to use this more general term "allergy" when discussing test results.

First it's important to know that allergy testing is a safe procedure. Allergy testing began around 1910, and techniques have been refined over the century since those early days, when samples of ragweed were pulverized, boiled, and sterilized, and small amounts were injected into patients. Unfortunately, there were no standards then, and several patients died. In the mid-1950s, England banned all types of allergy testing because of its high risk. From the 1950s to the 1980s, an additional seventeen patient deaths were recorded in the English literature. This was a mortality rate seemingly isolated to Great Britain because most physicians in England were using non-standardized raw ragweed pollen. They had no knowledge or control of potency. Thankfully, this old type of test material is no longer in use, and many common allergens are now standardized.

Modern *skin testing* includes intradermal tests and patch tests.

Intradermal testing can be done by either the prick method or by injection of a tiny amount of allergen under the skin. (Scratch tests, one of the old methods of skin testing, were found to be essentially worthless, and are now condemned by all allergy academies.) *Patch tests* are useful for the diagnosis of metal allergies and for sensitivity to some drugs or chemicals. Patch testing involves placing a small amount of the suspected allergen material, such as a piece of latex glove, under a Band-Aid and holding it against the skin for 24 hours to see if a rash develops. A rash would suggest a contact allergy — in this example, a contact allergy to latex.

Skin testing	Blood Testing
~~Scratch~~	Total IgE
Patch	Specific IgE
Prick	RAST ®
Intradermal	Thabest ®
	IgG

Figure 6: Types of Skin and Blood Tests

If your pediatrician or ENT surgeon doesn't do allergy testing, but refers you to an allergist, you should understand, as should your doctor, that whomever he or she uses for referrals would determine the kind of testing you would get. If your family physician or pediatrician refers you or your child to a *pediatric- or internal medicine–trained "general" allergist,* you'll most likely get prick testing and have less than a 30 percent chance of diagnosing your allergies. I base this number on the fact that I've kept track of hundreds of patients who've come from the general allergists to my practice, and have compared our results. Because of the low sensitivity of prick testing, despite nearly all being tested, fewer than 30 percent of the patients from these allergists had their allergy diagnosis confirmed by positive tests, despite having classic symptoms. More perplexing is that allergy shots, or immunotherapy, was recommended to fewer than 20 percent of those who were found positive to their prick testing — contrary to their own guidelines.

It is important for you to understand what a doctor is looking for when he or she does a specific allergy test. The major goals of any allergy testing are first, to find out whether or not you *have* allergies, and second, to find out what strength of allergy mixture is safe to use when you start treatment. Let us look at exactly how the two testing methods are similar but different. Hopefully this will not be too technical.

PRICK TESTING

General allergists, as members of the American Academy of Allergy, Asthma and Immunology (AAAAI), *use prick testing for their initial diagnosis.* They may occasionally add additional intradermal testing by injection, which will be explained shortly. General allergists still predominantly deal with severe asthmatics, so they use prick testing because it is extremely dilute, at approximately one part allergen to 50,000 parts sterile water, or 1:50,000.

With the prick test method, the allergen is introduced by dipping a small needle into a solution containing an antigen and pricking the skin. Understand that although prick testing is technically a form of intradermal testing (that is, placing the antigen into the skin layer itself), it is never referred to as intradermal testing. *When I use the term intradermal testing, I am referring to the injection method.*

When doctors conduct prick tests, they are looking for bumps, or "wheals," to be produced on the skin that are "greater than two plus" in size. Usually this means greater than or equal to three millimeters in diameter. The prick test makes a small, medium, or large wheal that is considered "1+," "2+," "3+," or "4+." The larger the wheal, the more sensitive you are and so doctors will begin to treat you at a lower amount of allergen. *Note that this grading system is totally subjective, in that it is not measured by any standardized unit — mm, inches, or what?* As noted, the reaction from the prick test produces a bump that is measured and rated on a scale of "1+" to "4+." Since this is not a precise measurement, prick testing introduces a great deal of variability. Usually a one or two plus is considered negative or nonreactive.

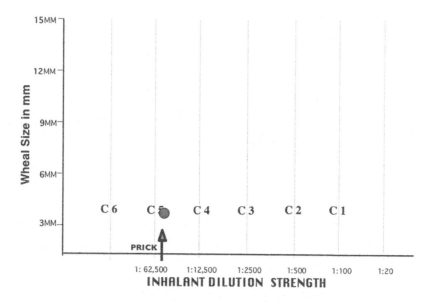

Figure 7: Prick Test – Single point produced with single intradermal at 1:50,000

Most general allergists put on just a single test at a very low dose for each allergen. (Figure 7) Obviously, if the patient needed a somewhat stronger concentration before he would react, the general allergists would miss the diagnosis unless they tested at a higher concentration of allergen. Therefore, when faced with a negative prick test the general allergist may do an intradermal test at a concentration of 1:1,000 (Figure 8). This is their attempt to try to adapt to the more accurate testing methods used by ENT allergists.

In contrast to this straight line, the ENT allergy testing procedure produces a dose-response curve so as to determine a reaction at any strength of allergen exposure, as described below.

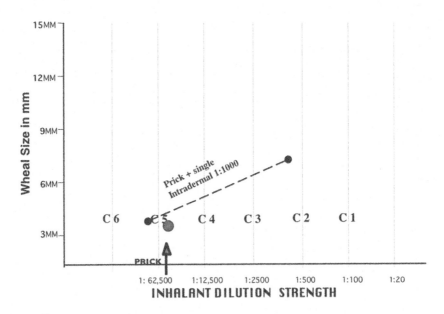

Figure 8: Prick plus extra intradermal at 1:1000

Because of the minute allergen doses delivered by the prick method, these tests do avoid major reactions, *but also miss the majority of allergies in people with less severe disease than life-threatening asthma.* Prick testing at such minute allergen levels will diagnose fewer than 50 percent of true allergy in patients with runny noses, and less than 20 percent of patients with chronic middle ear disease. Patients with these two diseases must be tested at higher strengths, and that involves intradermal testing by injection. This is detailed shortly.

I am aware that almost all research on allergy is based on prick testing, so why do I find it so unsatisfactory? Prick testing is very specific in that a positive test really means the patient has allergies. It just does not find *all* the patients who have allergy. The shortcoming of prick testing is that it is 40 to 50 percent falsely negative.[17] That is, it may miss real allergy 40 to 50 percent of the time. That may be all right for a research tool, but it does not help you, the patient, if it misses half the patients with middle ear or sinus disease who has allergies the test does not pick up. It is like relying on an air traffic controller to tell us when he *sees* a plane coming rather than using a more sensitive test like radar. A lot of planes will go undetected, possibly with dire consequences.

INTRADERMAL ALLERGY TESTING

ENT allergists prefer intradermal testing which involves introducing a small amount of allergen (or antigen) material under the skin. The intradermal testing I describe here is when a *precisely measured* amount of an allergen is injected under the skin to form a small bump, or wheal. Prick testing and intradermal testing are very different in both their methodology and precision, and therefore differ in their results.

TESTING FOR INHALANTS, MOLDS, OR FOODS

The object of true intradermal testing is *to determine precisely how much* dust, dog, cat, or grass pollen antigen is required to produce a reaction in a person. Once that reaction occurs, the body's response is the same: a release of histamine, lots of congestion or sneezing, and/or ear fluid, but with the small volume used in either testing it is rare to produce more than local redness or a bump at the test site.

ENT Allergists use intradermal testing almost exclusively. The ENT allergy academy (American Academy of Otolaryngologic Allergy = AAOA) teaches all of us to do our testing exactly alike. In contrast to the non-standardized prick test, ENT allergists define as positive any reaction that produces a wheal that is at least two millimeters larger than a "control" of normal saline or glycerin used to dilute the antigen. (Figure 9) The size of the reaction is measured with a standardized gauge and recorded.

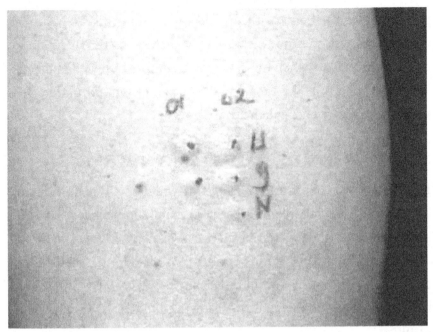

Figure 9: Skin testing.
Controls: H = histamine, G = glycerine, N = normal saline control.

Besides the advantage of measuring exactly how much dust, cat dander, or pollen allergen is introduced, we also test at different concentrations, which have been standardized throughout the country for sixty years. Intradermal testing by an ENT allergist begins at safe antigen doses similar to an initial prick test, but then proceeds in a much more precise manner.

First, and most importantly, the amount of allergen injected is precise and measured at 0.01 cubic centimeters regardless of the allergen or dilution. The allergen is tested in a series of strengths, each one being five times stronger than the last. The testing begins at the sixth dilution or concentration #6 (C-6). This dilution is 1:312,500, actually much weaker than a prick test of 1:50,000. The dilutions continue up four to five steps, until concentration of C-5 = 1:62,500, C-4 = 1:12,500, C-3 = 1:2,500, or C-2 = 1:500 is reached. (Figure 10) Just like the prick test, intradermal testing will produce a single bump or wheal. This wheal is compared to a standard of 0.01 cubic centimeters of both histamine and normal saline solution tested on that patient. The histamine is considered a "positive control," and must always be larger than the test with normal saline. [18]

Therefore, rather than having a graph of patient response with only a single point on it (Figure 7) or a straight line (Figure 8) and trying to *guess* how gently or severely a patient will react, the ENT allergist produces a graph curve indicating test responses at a minimum of three to six strengths (Figure 10).

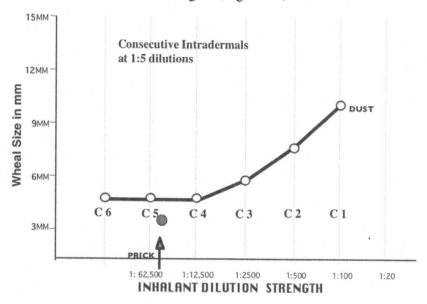

Figure 10: Curve produced by intradermal testing at multiple strengths.

Using a method that produces a curve can accommodate and diagnose allergy safely in ultra-sensitive, "brittle" patients (meaning more easily triggered to an over-response) like severe asthmatics. We ENT allergists can also diagnose allergy in patients with chronic middle ear disease who generally are much less sensitive. The graphs in Figure 11 and Figure 12 show some examples of the response using multiple stronger dilutions produced by this testing method on various patients.

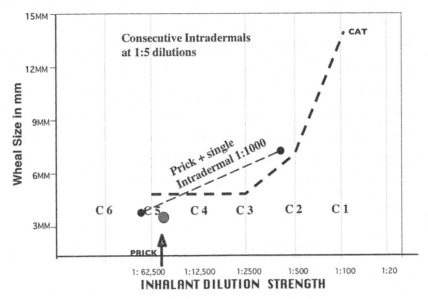

Figure ll: Curve of Hyper Response to Cat

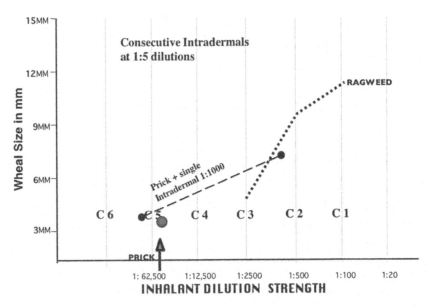

Figure l2: Curve of Hyper Response to Ragweed

By definition, to be considered significant or "positive" the response to an allergen must produce a wheal that is at least two millimeters larger than that produced by a control dose of normal saline. If the patient is very sensitive, he or she will be positive at the sixth or fifth dilution (C-6 or C-5), about equal to a prick test. However, most patients with allergic rhinitis or otitis media will not be positive until the higher concentrations at dilutions of C-3 or C-2, (Appendix C: circled results in Figures B,D,F) so the diagnosis of all these patients would be missed by the general allergist.

What does the testing mean? What use is the testing?

Two areas of interest in testing are: First, at what strength does the patient begin to show a reaction? Looking back at our testing examples: this may be point C-5 in Figure 10 and equal to the prick test. Or the first reaction may not occur until concentration C-3 or C-2. And second, how rapidly does the patient react to the increasing concentrations? As the concentration increases five-fold, one would anticipate a general progression in the size of the wheal. What is most important is to know whether the patient reacts in the gentle progressive manner (5mm, 7mm, 9mm) seen in Figure 10, or with a slope that looks like a rocket just took off (5mm, 9mm, 13mm) as seen in Figure 11 or 12, which would indicate extreme sensitivity. These patients must be treated more carefully, and your doctor, if he or she were an ENT allergist, would understand that.

Again, should this response begin at the second, C-2, or even weaker C-3 concentration, these patients would not have been identified by the prick test at all — the doctor would totally miss your diagnosis. Furthermore, that single test would not give any indication as to how quickly and severely this particular patient might react.

Besides being safer, intradermal testing simply gives more information and picks up allergy among patients who are not severe asthmatics but have only "low-sensitivity disease." By this I mean that their **total IgE**, which is a measure of the severity of their allergy, is really quite low. (We will discuss IgE in a little more detail in the next section under "Other types of testing.") The average total IgE among patients with chronic middle ear disease ranges from five to eighty, whereas the average total IgE among asthmatics is over 100, with some reaching levels of 5,000! The general allergist, in all fairness, deals with these more "brittle" patients, and so uses a technique that usually detects allergy among asthmatics, but almost always misses allergy among patients with chronic middle ear disease or those of you who have only "a little runny nose."

The obvious advantage to the intradermal injection method over the prick method is that the absolute amount of testing material injected is measured precisely each time. This leads to consistency of results and reproducibility. There are multiple studies that show a great deal of variability in results using the prick test — as much as 50 percent — no better than a coin toss! Prick testing depends on each testing person's methods and how much liquid is picked up by the little prick device (which is similar to the lancet needle used to prick your finger for a simple blood test at the doctor's office).

Medicare did an audit of allergy charts in 2001 and found that prick testing results from the majority of general allergists were reported differently. Most showed no scale at all, no controls, and there was a lack of standardization of what constituted a positive test.

(See **Appendix C** for a comparison of test results from general allergists and an ENT allergist for the same patient.)

ENT allergists use objective scientific methods throughout their testing procedures. They do not rely on subjective observations such as "it looked like a two-plus reaction."

Remember the mousetrap analogy I used earlier? I like to compare the mucous membrane to a mousetrap. If the mousetrap has a stiff spring, even an aggressive mouse won't trigger it, but if the mousetrap has a hair trigger, it will snap at the slightest jiggling. Once it does snap, the reaction in either situation is the same: BANG! Sometimes allergic people are triggered by a tiny bit of allergen, and sometimes it takes a whole lot before they react. Prick testing only finds the people with a hair trigger and misses the others.

So why am I so evangelical about this? Because:

Treatment is based on test results.

Adult, age 22

Dr. Hurst:

I am a 22-year-old female and I have had chronic ear infections or so thought to be for 10 years. I have been tested for allergies and found that I am allergic to almost everything outside. I get allergy shots once a month, take Claritin-D 24Hour, and use Nasonex. This seems to help my ears more than any of the medications I've ever used. So my question is, could my ear infections have been caused by my allergies with the outside? I've been to an ENT many times and he always wants to put tubes in my ears. I've had tubes so many times I'm beginning to think that my eardrum is nothing but scar tissue. I would greatly appreciate hearing what you have to say.

Thanks,

Mancine

Reply:

Dear Mancine,

You have already discovered that allergies are a major source of the cause of your ear disease, but still you are not 100% better. Most likely you are seeing a classic allergist—someone who does not test for or treat many MOLDS or FOODS.

The fact that you are not better despite the shots means that they are missing something in the treatment set. Even so, adults with this long history are difficult and your allergies keep changing every few years, so you may have to be skin tested again—by an ENT allergist.

Good luck,
Dr. Hurst

IMMUNOTHERAPY

Immunotherapy involves giving repeated tiny amounts of the allergen to which you have reacted until you are "desensitized." The initial amount or "dose" of allergen is approximated based on the size of the test response. For the general allergist that may be based solely on a single prick test "dot." (Figure 7) If that initial amount is too large, you could have a bad reaction. If that dose begins at too small an amount, it might take years to be desensitized. Often a general allergist will tell you it will take two years to bring you up to an adequate amount of allergen in the desensitization shots so you are maintained at a full treatment level.

This is in contrast to the ENT allergist, who knows more precisely where to start based on the curve of responses to three or four tested strengths of an allergen. (Figures 10, 11, 12) He/she will therefore usually have a patient up to a full maintenance dose within four months. Because the single prick does not tell the doctor how quickly or slowly you will react when you get their shots, general allergists expect perhaps10 percent of their patients to have some sort of reaction (usually only mild itching, sneezing or wheezing) right in the office as they increase the allergy shot dosage. They simply don't know if you are going to react quickly or slowly. ENT allergists are also prepared for severe reactions, but they happen in less than one in 40,000 injections. [19]

I've seen letters from general allergists to patients and their referring primary care physicians discouraging the use of allergy shots altogether. I think that at a subconscious level the allergists and their staffs are leery of patients having significant reactions in their offices and therefore wary of giving allergy shots. This thinking is reinforced by the position of the general allergists' medical academy (the American Academy of Asthma, Allergy, and Immunology), who's guidelines state that all patients must wait in the doctor's office for at least thirty minutes following an allergy shot.

Also, general allergists never allow patients to take their shots at home, while ENT allergists do allow their nonasthmatic patients to do their shots at home after reaching a maintenance dose, as it has been proven safe. Safety is our greatest concern. I published a paper in 1999 that looked at the reactions after giving 1.4 million shots in over 40 ENT offices throughout the country. We showed that receiving an allergy shot from an ENT allergist is thirty times safer than taking a penicillin pill.[19] Allergy shots, or immunotherapy, like anything else in medicine, are of course not *absolutely* guaranteed to be safe, yet there has never been a death reported among patients treated by a member of the ENT allergists' academy. I will discuss immunotherapy in Chapter Ten.

BLOOD TESTS

Allergies can also be diagnosed by a variety of blood testing techniques. Basically each of the blood tests measures specific *immunoglobulin E*, or *IgE*. These are antibodies the body produces in response to exposure to an allergenic foreign substance such as dust, pollen, or animal dander. IgE triggers the inflammatory response that is responsible for the classic allergic symptoms — sneezing, congestion, runny nose, and middle ear fluid.

The methodologies of the different blood tests are similar, but sometimes the results are very different, along the lines of hitting a drum with your fist vs. your palm. Each produces slightly different sounds depending on how the drum was struck. Similarly, each allergy laboratory strives to develop a method that is more sensitive so it can diagnose allergy in patients with minimal sensitivity. As the tests detect lower and lower levels of sensitivity, sometimes what is called "background noise" will produce a false positive test. There is always a balance required between increasing the sensitivity and avoiding a false positive test. It's a bit like trying to see in the dark without making the light too bright — the more you turn the lights down, the harder it is to see, and sometimes what you think you're seeing is something altogether different. You may even see things that aren't really there — a "false positive" sighting.

Almost all allergy blood tests are called *RAST tests;* RAST stands for *radioallerosorbent test*. Technically, however, RAST, per se, is no longer used because the "R" stands for radioactive. Labs no longer want radioactive materials around — so the technology has evolved, but the acronym RAST is still used even though most labs run ImmunoCAP®, developed in 1991, which has since replaced it.

All physicians have had allergy patients who they were absolutely convinced had allergy, yet when they drew a standard blood test it came back negative. In these cases, there is a disconnect between the physician's clinical judgment and the lab test results. Yet somehow we doctors tend to rely more heavily on the test results than on our own understanding of the patient's disease.

I have found that the most accurate blood test is called THABEST®. It seems to have the best correlation with intradermal skin tests.[20] In my search for a test to use for my own patients, I ran a comparison study. I looked at 27 patients with chronic middle ear disease and measured their reactions to standard RAST blood tests, intradermal testing (IDT), and THABEST testing. In patients who were very allergic and had high IgE levels, the RAST agreed perfectly with the IDT test. When the patients were less allergic, as indicated by lower total IgE scores, the RAST reported false negatives, or missed the diagnosis 86 percent of the time as compared to skin testing. On the other hand, the THABEST agreed with the intradermal testing 92 percent of the time. (It is important to note that RAST/ Immuno-CAP® testing may be useful for pollens and dust, yet it picks up fewer than 50 percent of patients with mold allergies, and fewer than 20 percent of patients with general food allergies. (The exception is life threatening allergens like latex, shrimp and peanut, for which RAST is reliable.) If your physician thinks that you have allergies and the results of the RAST test he/she ordered to diagnose what is causing your sinusitis, asthma or ear disease comes back negative, than you need to insist that he/she use a different method to confirm his/her clinical judgment.

[Note: Because of Health Maintenance Organization insurance, state insurance plans, and Medicare contracts, coupled with terrific marketing, all blood tests your doctor orders will be done by a lab that only uses some type of RAST/ ImmunoCAP testing. THABEST has to be ordered specifically from the only lab that does it. Its inventor lost his original testing to a large lab that bought him out and then shelved the technology in favor of the RAST technology they were already marketing. So he reinvented the THABEST, got around his own patent, and no longer trusts larger labs with running the test. It reminds me of how Firestone, Ford and Rockefeller (Standard Oil) got together and bought up all the railroads so they could tear up the tracks and eliminate competition for that new invention — the automobile.]

One obvious advantage of the blood tests is that they are much easier and take less time, especially when testing little children. I always use a THABEST in children under four rather than subject them to intradermal skin testing.

Thus, my conclusion after doing comparative testing is that the only accurate, reliable blood test that compares favorably to skin testing is a THABEST micro Eliza test. It is the only blood test accurate for children and for testing for mold allergies. (You should know, I have no association with the company.) Even with a positive THABEST, I like to confirm results in adults with intradermal testing. I do use the RAST to test for latex, peanut, and shellfish allergies.

A general allergist may argue that testing at the higher strengths used for intradermal testing gives false information. Though theoretically possible, there is not a single comparative study to support that assertion. Furthermore, when my ear patients were treated for all their "false positive" antigens – they resolved. There are, on the contrary, dozens of studies that show that using the low concentrations of prick testing misses more than half the cases of true allergy and therefore is inferior to intradermal testing.

Other studies show that immunotherapy is indicated for patients with asthma and allergic rhinitis,[3] as well as for patients with chronic middle ear fluid who are diagnosed with "low-sensitivity disease" but are indeed allergic when challenged with the actual allergen. These patients also are cured with allergy immunotherapy based on that testing.

In my recent study[21] we found that among those whose ear disease resolved on immunotherapy, 42 percent of the allergens had positive skin reactions only at a high concentration of C-2 or C-1. Prick testing alone (equal to a low test concentration of C-4) would have discovered only 10 percent of the allergens in patients with chronic effusion. Therefore, when it comes to skin testing, I rely completely on the intradermal method. In some states, insurance companies will not pay for intradermal testing unless prick testing has been done first. You can see why it is crucial to choose the kind of physician you want to do your testing if you want to know for sure that they will actually *detect* allergy if there *is* allergy. Deciding that you want intradermal skin testing has great significance in your choice of what kind of allergy specialist you will want to see.

The only way to guarantee that you'll have intradermal testing done is to see an ENT allergist. As stated earlier, this is a physician trained by either the American Academy of Otolaryngic Allergy (AAOA), the Pan American Allergy Society (PAAS) or the American Academy of Environmental Medicine (ACEM). In Appendix D, I provide information to help you locate the right specialist.

Now that we understand how testing is done, it is important for your allergist to consider what types of things you may be allergic to: dust, pollen, molds, or foods.

« 8 »

TESTING FOR MOLD AND FOOD ALLERGIES

*W*hat am I allergic to? You may be allergic to inhalants, molds, and/or foods. It is important that you and your doctor understand which type of allergen you think you might be bothered by or sensitive to. *Inhalants* include anything that can float through the air and be inhaled, such as dust, dander from cats, dogs, or other animals, and pollens from trees, grass, ragweed, goldenrod, or other plants. These are most easily identified through intradermal testing or blood tests, as described in the previous chapter.

Testing for *molds* can be a little more difficult than for inhalants. Molds may present both as inhalants and as foods. (Later I will explain some of the intricacies.) As for blood tests, the RAST testing for molds is about 50 percent accurate; the THABEST testing is about 85 percent accurate as compared to intradermal testing for the same mold in the same individual. (Remember, *when I use the term intradermal testing, I am referring to the injection method,* wherein a *precisely measured* amount of the allergen is injected under the skin to raise a small bump called a wheal.)

MOLDS AND FOODS

Allergy to foods and molds is a confusing and complicated topic. Much of the confusion is the result of academic arrogance and another of the semantic word-game discussions by doctors as to whether or not a reaction to a food is a classic "allergic response" involving IgE, or whether the reaction involves a separate, non-IgE mediated allergic pathway, or whether it is an "idiosyncratic" reaction particular to that patient alone. None of these semantic distinctions matter to you, the patient. *The real question is whether or not — because of its chemical mechanism or toxic byproduct or whatever its ability to cause an allergic reaction — a specific mold or food causes a true antigen-antibody response which gives you symptoms. In other words, does it make you sick?*

What is important is that your body responds to exposure to that food or mold in such a way that your head becomes congested or you have other allergic symptoms. What do you care about the technical mechanism?

These kinds of word-games come from the same kind of medical arrogance that physicians used when they refused to wash their hands for years after Semmelweis found in 1847 that it reduced deaths of pregnant women by over 80 percent. [It used to be, in old Germany, that surgeons would do a leg amputation, for example, wipe their hands on their long white coats, and then go to the delivery ward. The death rate for women who delivered babies under these conditions was 13 percent. Semmelweis said, "Wash your hands." and this reduced the rate to 2 percent. But that was thirty years before they knew that bacteria existed, so it made no sense to them. Those doctors didn't understand, so they refused to *believe* the science that proved they were endangering their patients. (http://en.wikipedia.org/wiki/Ignaz_Semmelweis)]

General allergists may think they are better scientists than ENT allergists (they do know more immunology), but they are frequently paralyzed into inaction and won't treat the patients in front of them with immunotherapy until they have "more studies." ENT allergists are more pragmatic and tend to use what has been clinically proven to work and is safe— and wait for the "science" to catch up with their empirical, practical "art of medicine."

INHALANT MOLDS

Mold allergies are perhaps the most significant "hidden" cause of allergies. You easily connect petting a cat and suddenly sneezing, but you never see the mold. In my experience, molds are more allergenic than animals or ragweed, in that more people are allergic to them. Almost 90 percent of my otitis patients tested positive to molds. In a study of school children almost 40 percent of those who tested positive to molds had asthma or wheezing. [22]

Molds are interesting because we can be exposed to them either by breathing them as inhalants floating in the air or by eating them. Yeast is simply a one-cell mold. Molds can reproduce in several ways. They can produce thread-like arms or buds, which are called hyphae. They can also produce spores. You may have seen this if you've opened a puffball in the woods. Molds will release their spores just before, during, or immediately after a rain. So when a patient comes in and tells a doctor she can tell by her head congestion when the weather is going to change, she is absolutely right. *She is not crazy. It is a doctor who doesn't understand mold biology who is actually the ignorant one.*

Patients with mold allergies will often have problems in the spring or fall in the Northeast because these are our two rainy seasons. April showers bring May flowers but they also bring the molds. Similarly, after the leaves fall off the trees in autumn, they sit in the woods and rot — releasing a huge mold load. Mold-allergic people raking the leaves off their lawns in the fall often get congested because they have simply raked up a lot of mold.

Another classic situation is the patient who complains that every time he mows the lawn he gets congested. He's not allergic to grass, because grass only pollinates in the spring. To be allergic to a plant, you have to be allergic to the pollen of that plant, but most lawns in suburbia never pollinate. What is really happening is that after the grass is cut, the grass clippings rot. The next week, when the allergic person mows the lawn again, blowing the now moldy, rotten grass clippings up into the air with that fan we call a rotary lawn mower, he becomes congested with his ears all stuffed up.

We are not really sure if people are allergic to the cell wall of the mold or to parts of its interior cellular structure. Molds grow and change depending on the amount of humidity they are exposed to. This makes it very difficult to make a good allergen serum for a specific mold because so much depends on its growing conditions and what parts of the mold cell, or coating, or spore the laboratory uses to make the allergen sample. Each mold will have dozens of separate antigens. Fortunately, a great number of them are similar in a variety of mold species. It is the same as with humans: we all have the same basic structure, but all look very different.

Of the major molds such as *Alternaria*, *Hormodendrum*, and *Aspergillus*, there may be 50,000 species of each. You can see how complicated the problem is. The general allergist usually only tests for these three molds because that's where all the scientific research has been concentrated. On the other hand, we know that there are thirty or more significant molds that different people have commonly been shown to be reactive to. Most ENT allergists will check for ten to thirty molds, depending on the environmental conditions where their practice is located.

MOLD TOXINS

In addition to allergens from the mold itself or from yeast, molds also give off toxins. Toxic molds are an increasing problem in our environment, especially after floods and hurricanes. In the 1970s and 1980s, it was popular to make homes airtight with vapor barriers in the walls and ceilings. This kept the heat in and saved on heating bills and air-conditioning costs. Unfortunately, a very tight house does not breathe. If indoor humidity gets above 60 percent, mold grows on everything. Sometimes in the winter in a tight house, there will actually be condensation on the windows inside and mold growing on the windowsills.

Sometimes buildings with poor ventilation produce conditions called "sick building syndrome." It is thought that this may be from the toxins released by the molds growing in the heating and air-handling duct system. In the mold-sensitive person, it is most likely the overexposure to a huge concentration of the mold itself that triggers symptoms. Cleaning air ducts and installing good filters in the ductwork, or placing stand-alone filters, are effective ways to minimize inhalant molds. HEPA filters work best. All the variations with ionizers, etc., in my opinion add unnecessary, unproven gadgets at additional cost.

Another group of patients I see regularly are teachers who suffer from a worsening of their allergy symptoms when school opens up in the fall. Schools are notorious because the contractor with the lowest bid builds them. In New England, despite our snowy winters, schools often have flat roofs, so there are a lot of school buildings with leaky roofs. Or classes are taught in basements, which suffer from condensation and are moldy. Some schools have carpeted floors, and when the children come in from recess with their wet boots, the carpet is saturated, and this also leads to a mold problem. Often, the only practical solution is to get out of the building.

If you walk into a room and it smells musty, and you are allergic to molds, you had better get out. (If you walk into a room and smell smoke, it's time to get out because where there's smoke, there's fire. Well, as far as your body is concerned, that mold in the room is fire.) This problem has become so serious in schools and some homes because of poor construction or flooding, that most homeowner insurance policies have limited or completely eliminated coverage for mold damage. Short of running away, allergy immunotherapy provides significant relief for the employee who simply cannot change jobs or the homeowner who cannot afford to move.

"BRAIN FOG," ECZEMA AND OTHER STRANGE REACTIONS

Patients with mold allergy may present not just with classic head congestion, but also with unexpected mood swings. Men get aggressive and women get bitchy. (One of my college age fellows told me that he avoids pizza because the cheese will make him pick fights.)

Patients with mold allergy often complain of fatigue, and what I call "brain fog." When in the moldy environment, these patients have problems concentrating. They make lists, then lose them; they go upstairs and forget what they went upstairs for. They have some days when they are thinking clearly and other days when they are in a "brain fog." They may get confused when they go downstairs to the basement to work in a shop or to do the laundry or when they turn on the heat or air conditioner in the car. The air conditioner is simply a condenser and water forms in the hoses in the automobile, mold grows, and with the ignition system on mold is blown into the passenger compartment. Here again, they are exposed to mold-laden air.

The severity of the brain fog experience depends on the mold exposure. Patients who have experienced these symptoms but haven't connected them to allergies are deeply relieved when I reassure them that these are not signs of early dementia, and that they aren't "going crazy."

An unusual manifestation of mold allergy is eczema – but in unusual places. This is not like the classic dry skin of the arms or legs. These patients will instead have red, broken out areas on their fingers or palms and particularly the back of the wrists or knuckles. Another presentation is redness and sometimes puffiness of the mustache area or upper eyelids, fissures in the corner of the nose or lips; redness and/or scaling in the hollow of the ear just outside the ear canal, often with extension down under the earlobe, sometimes again with cracking or fissure and sometimes involving the greater part of the outer ear. A significant percentage of these, if women, have a chronic inflammation in the area of the vulva and even vaginitis not limited to times when they are taking antibiotics. Of course these first need to be seen by a dermatologist, but if they throw up their hands and really do not know what it is, or what to do – in my experience these are classic signs of mold food allergy. Many will only resolve with a strict mold elimination diet. (See Appendix A.)

Ricky, age 4½

Ricky was brought in by his mother because of his recurrent ear infections. This would happen mainly in the spring and fall but often the fluid would not clear for three months. In addition he had severe eczema. His face cheeks were red and sometimes his hands would break out so badly that his mother would keep his hands wrapped in gauze mittens to keep the cortisone cream on them – even in preschool! He had been seen multiple times by a dermatologist. He was also a mouth breather, had a continual runny nose, congestion and was thought to have ADHD because he seemed to have a lot of hyperactivity. His IgE was very elevated at 412.

His skin testing was done in the operating room while he was asleep while I put in his first set of tubes and removed his adenoids. He was positive to dust, dog, grass, weeds and at least 10 molds. He was also positive for wheat and cheese. Because it's impossible for his mother to withhold dairy products and wheat from this young child (with 4 brothers and sisters) we put him on sublingual immunotherapy for those two foods as well as for the dust, dog, grass and molds. We also put him on a full mold elimination diet. Within four months the eczema on his face totally cleared. He no longer needed to bandage his hands as they were 90% improved.

I followed him intermittently for five years and at times he would have breakthroughs if he got into too much cheese. He never needed a second set of tubes because he no longer had any ear infections. His grades improved. I last saw him when he was 10 and he still had to be careful to not eat too much cheese or mold containing foods but otherwise he was doing well. I saw his mother years later and she told me that he's totally healthy, finished college and has gone into TV broadcasting. His ears are fine!

For patients with chronic middle ear disease, there is very little day-to-day fluctuation of the symptom of ear fullness, but over half of these patients also have nasal allergies and head congestion and many have accompanying brain fog and/or eczema as described above. All are clues that they may be mold-allergic.

Adult, age 62

I first met Clarence when he was 58. He was a classic hard-working Mainer and came down to see me from two hours "down East." His left ear was perforated 20 years ago by a piece of welding slag. That left ear seemed to drain three to five times a year the last 20 years. He was sent to see me because the current episode of drainage had persisted for about four months and it seemed that he had a fungal infection in that ear.

The right ear had no perforation but he developed fluid in it at least two to four times a year and it might take a month or so for his hearing to return to normal. His audiogram revealed a 20 to 25 dB hearing loss in each ear.

Because of the persistent fluid in the right ear I thought that allergy must have something to do with his problem. Intradermal skin testing found him allergic to dust, molds and ragweed. He began allergy immunotherapy and within four months both ears cleared up.

I also noted that after a year and a half on his shots *the perforation of his left ear which he had had for 20 years had closed spontaneously*!

Two years into treatment he came back unexpectedly because he developed fluid again in his right ear. This seemed to have happened suddenly while he had spent a weekend cleaning out an old house that had been abandoned for a few years. It was full of molds. His mold allergy filled his ears again. It was interesting that he had no other target organ for his allergies besides his middle ears. He never got congested.

"MOLDY" FOODS

Mold foods are a special topic. Of course you don't think of eating moldy foods, but basically anything that tastes good these days has been fermented. About a third of my patients allergic to mold particles in the air are also affected by mold in their foods. As already stated, yeasts are single-celled molds, so raised, yeasty breads, cinnamon buns, and tasty donuts are moldy-food culprits. Among vinegar-containing foods, pickles, salad dressings, mustard, catsup, and mayonnaise head the list. Cheeses of all kinds have mold in them, as do sour cream and flavored yogurts, dried fruits, and, of course, wine and beer. Safe foods are plain, non-processed meats, vegetables, and fruits.

Sugar cravers have a problem because sugars feed the natural mold in our gut. Our digestive tract is just a long tube of skin where food goes in one end and plops out the other. Inside are yeast (*Candida*) and a bacterium (*E. coli*). They both are essential for digestion. But if you get antibiotics in excess, the *E. coli* gets killed and you get a *Candida* overgrowth, or "yeast infection." You feel terrible and lethargic. (Sometimes women even get a vaginal yeast infection.) If you are mold-sensitive and you eat too much sugar, the *Candida* inside your gut says, "Whoopee, dessert!" and explodes with more growth. You experience a sudden internal mold overload and get symptomatic. This is a common cause of congestion and fatigue in these patients, especially after meals. Recently, probiotics have gained popularity. They are really "good yeasts," such as *Acidophilus*, which are used to replace the killed *Candida* in your bowel. Many health food books feature information on them.

This book is not meant to be a thorough discussion of mold and food allergies, so I have listed in the appendix some references and sources for further information, as well as the handouts I use in my office that list foods to avoid as well as safe foods for maintaining a mold-elimination diet. Just remember, molds are as allergenic as dust or cats or pollen, but in addition to breathing them, you can also be exposed by eating mold-containing foods.

Food allergy is another controversial topic. Is it a true allergy or an "idiosyncratic reaction?" Food allergies can present with obvious rashes, asthma or life threatening anaphylaxis (peanuts, shrimp, nuts or antibiotics). Many of my allergy patients get congestion from some foods but a great many in addition have various gastro-intestinal symptoms: bloating, colic, diarrhea and cramps. Perhaps as many as a third of toddlers with chronic middle ear disease have been found to be allergic to a food.[12, 23]

Children

Hello Dr. Hurst,

I have three sons, each with a history of ear infections. Their ages are 4, 3, and 17 months. They all have had ear tubes placed. The first has had two sets and an adenoidectomy. He has allergies to environmental stuff and asthma.

My second child had terrible ear infections and had tubes placed when he was 2-1/2. He continued to have the ear infections even with the tubes. The tubes became blocked and he was going to get yet another set of tubes, when I decided to take him off dairy completely. No whey, casein, milk, etc. His ear infections cleared up completely and his tubes started functioning again. No doctor will confirm this "miracle" because of the dairy.

I am convinced it is because of the dairy. He was skin tested for milk protein. It came back negative, but I know those tests are not always accurate. Is this allergy?

Jennifer G.

Reply:

Absolutely!

Food allergies are fascinating, but difficult to diagnose. Your response can be immediate or delayed for days, making it very difficult to diagnose exactly what the culprit food might be. Testing for food allergies offers the greatest challenge. Only about 20 percent of true food allergies involve the IgE system, and therefore the RAST/ImmunoCAP blood test can only be expected to pick up a small percentage of truly food-allergic patients. In my experience, intradermal skin testing for foods will pick up a true food allergy in 50 to 60 percent of patients. Technically, the skin test measures more than simply the IgE response, and that is why it is better for discovering allergy to foods (as well as to molds) than blood tests of any sort. Regardless of what test is used for food, I consider them all to be *merely indicators*.

All positive food testing should be confirmed. You must make sure that a particular food actually causes symptoms. This is done by a simple *seven-day elimination-challenge diet*. If a patient tests positive to milk, I have them eliminate all dairy products for a week, avoiding all milk, ice cream, cheese, and yogurt. This puts them in a hypersensitive state. I then have them overload themselves with a challenge of dairy products. If symptoms such as nasal congestion or GI symptoms improve during the elimination week, and especially if the symptoms recur upon challenge, then the patient knows he or she is truly allergic to that particular food. It should be avoided.

Here is an example of how this can work:

Child, age 2

Dear Doctor Hurst,

We have a 2-year-old daughter who contracted her first ear infection this December. The first antibiotic she was placed on was Amoxicillin. She immediately had an allergic reaction (swelling of the face and a slight rash). She was then placed on every other antibiotic known to man to try and clear up her ear infection. She would show improvement for the first 8 days or so, however, usually prior to the end of the medication or immediately following,she would get another infection.

We finally agreed to put tubes in her ears. Her ear infection went away, but at her post-surgery checkup 10 days later she had tonsillitis. Following that, she again contracted another ear infection. After some debate, we decided to have both her tonsils and adenoids removed and another set of tubes (titanium). This procedure cleared her up for approximately 6 weeks. On June 8th she developed a sinus infection and her ears drained pus. She was placed on Ceftin (which seems to work best for her) and she cleared up. On June 30th she began to show signs again and she was slightly congested, but not enough to warrant yet another antibiotic. On July 31st she developed another ear infection.

My husband and I are at our wit's end. She does seem to have allergies, as her nose really starts running when she is outside, especially if it is windy. The ENT and the pediatrician are both suggesting a CAT scan to make sure she does not have mastoiditis, and to check out her sinuses. She seems to show no signs of any hearing loss (both the ENT and pediatrician agree) and is a very happy child who does not even seem bothered by all that is going on. As parents we survived the tubes, tonsils and adenoid removal, but now they are talking sinus surgery and we aren't sure what to think. What do you suggest?

Karen and Jeff

Reply:

Your doctors keep looking for another test to look for WHAT is happening and still do not look for WHY her ears keep getting infected or drain.

The infant or toddler with constant draining tubes almost always has food allergies. Do not worry—it was correct to put in the tubes, but the fact that they are steadily draining is a sign of allergy and almost always in toddlers it is to a food. First try to eliminate all her dairy products for a week—no milk, cheese, ice cream, or yogurt (water is wonderful—no one is allergic to it). Then, after 10 days—load her up! You cannot see what her ears do, but you can see what her nose does. See if the ear drainage—and runny nose—stops. Milk allergies account for 1/3 of the cases of draining ears in toddlers. If not that, then she needs a full blood evaluation — THABEST — for other foods, dust, etc.

2 weeks later:

Dear Dr. Hurst,

Thanks for your response. I took your advice and took her completely off of dairy. It has now been 13 days and not one runny nose, ear draining, etc. Mikayla is actually on her second set of tubes. I appreciate your web page. I find it interesting that my husband and I repeatedly asked her pediatrician and her ENT if we should take her off milk, and both insisted that since she was 2 and had never previously had any problems with dairy products that allergy could not possibly be the cause. So far we are infection free!

Thanks again!

« 9 »

TREATMENT CHOICES - THE 3 M'S

The universally accepted treatments for allergies consist of: 1) avoidance, 2) medication or pharmacotherapy, and 3) immuno-therapy. Remember my "3 M's" approach to allergy treatment? I summarize the options for my patients, and tell them they can:

> continue what they're doing and be *miserable*,
> *mask* their symptoms with medication, or
> *modify* their immune system with immunotherapy or allergy shots.

Avoidance makes the most sense and is the most obvious treatment choice. If you know that every time you pet a dog you have an asthma attack, it makes sense to avoid dogs. A great majority of patients are only allergic to one or two things, so avoidance works for them. However, I have found patients who have chronic middle ear disease (and I hope you are reading this book!) have allergies to half a dozen or more things, including inhalants, molds, and sometimes foods.

In fact, in the 1990s, my mentor, Dr. Venge, and I published studies[10, 23] involving over 250 of our patients with chronic middle ear disease and found that most patients (85.7 percent) were *pan allergic* (reactive to multiple allergens) to an average of nine allergens, including dust (94 percent), animals (47 percent), ragweed (67 percent), and molds (88 percent). Only ten percent were allergic solely to seasonal pollens. Therefore, if you have chronic allergic diseases such as asthma, sinusitis, or chronic middle ear effusion, adequate avoidance of all your allergens will be impossible.

A basic tenet of allergy therapy is the *total allergy load,* which refers to how many things you are exposed to simultaneously. The balance between sickness and health is like a seesaw. If you are allergic to ten things and they are all out of control, the seesaw is out of balance and you are very symptomatic. If you can get half of those allergens under control, your body can often manage the other half and the seesaw comes into balance and you feel fine.

Total Allergy Load

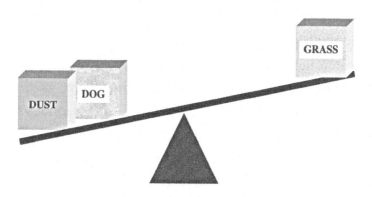

Figure 13: Total Allergy Load

Anything you can do to reduce your total allergy load by reducing exposure, such as dust proofing the house or avoiding areas you know make you sick, will help to reduce your allergy symptoms. That is why avoidance is such a powerful allergy management tool.

I've had several patients with severe sinus disease who have been so successful in reducing their total allergy load by addressing the dust in their houses with air filters and adequate bed and mattress covers, and by removing carpets to eliminate old molds and animal byproducts that they have been able to stop all allergy therapy and all medication.

MEDICATIONS

The most effective medications for allergy symptoms are antihistamines, anti-leukotrienes (a new class of drugs such as Singulair), and corticosteroids or prednisone. There is also a new anti-IgE medication (Xolair) which you need to know about. Remember, allergy simply means that you react abnormally to normal things around you: dust, animals, molds, pollens, or foods. After you have been exposed to an allergen, your body makes antibodies to it, and on re-exposure your body overreacts and releases histamine and a number of other chemicals that cause inflammation.

To stop the symptoms of allergic reactions, doctors prescribe "anti" histamines. Antihistamines sometimes help, as they are designed to block the effects of histamine. Antihistamines are very effective for nasal allergy, and most are also effective for itching and hives. Unfortunately, antihistamines provide almost no benefit for asthma or middle ear disease. The reason for this I will explain in *Chapter Eleven: To Your Doctor.*

Child

Dear Doctor Hurst:

    I've got an allergy kid that had constant ear infections (575 days on antibiotics) until I realized he was allergic to peanuts and soy (don't do beans anymore either). Didn't know he was allergic because his ears were almost the only problem he was showing besides a little runny nose. Occasional asthma if a cold went down into his chest. ENT said "no allergy" when I asked. NOT! Identified allergens (peanut butter sandwiches during the school year was the key) and since then, almost no more ear infections requiring antibiotics. I thought I was crazy with what I was seeing in his ear.

K. C.

But treating only the symptoms of the disease is like giving morphine to someone with appendicitis – they need it out. Furthermore, although television marketing tells us antihistamines are twice as good as using a "sugar pill," or placebo, they don't mention that only 20 percent of allergic people feel better on the sugar pill. Therefore, since antihistamines are "twice as good," *they may block 40 percent of the symptoms in the average allergic patient.* This means that *60 percent of allergic nasal symptoms do not respond to a particular antihistamine.* So it's no wonder that you may need to try several kinds until you get lucky and find one that works — maybe. That leaves you reaching for a decongestant.

Sudafed (pseudoephedrine) is a most effective decongestant. It sometimes helps open your nasal passages so you can breathe better, but at times it has a side effect in that it makes it difficult to sleep, or may cause rapid heartbeat. Guaifenesin (sold under the brand name Musinex) is considered a decongestant because it takes the pressure off your sinuses, but it does that by actually thinning the mucus. It has no cardiac side effects. Most drug companies make antihistamines in combination with pseudoephedrine.

Another major group of chemicals released by an allergic response are leukotrienes. These are similar to histamines in that they cause a lot of inflammation in the mucous membrane. Therefore anti-leukotrienes like Singulair can help. This newer class of medication has been available since about 2000. These medications were initially designed for asthmatics, but have been found to be helpful in one-third of patients with nasal symptoms. Theoretically, they might be of benefit early on in the patient with ear congestion due to allergies, but it has been shown that Singulair, like antihistamines, is ineffective in clearing fluid that has been present for more than a few weeks.[24]

There are no specific medications for all the other chemicals released in an allergic reaction except corticosteroids. Corticosteroids are the most potent medications available to treat allergic reactions to almost everything — including poison ivy, drug reactions, and out-of-control asthma attacks. The most common corticosteroid is prednisone. While useful and safe when taken for a short term situation, longterm or frequent refills of *oral* corticosteroids may lead to serious side effects and should be discussed with your physician.

There are also several kinds of corticosteroids used as inhalers both for asthma and chronic allergic nasal conditions. These are very effective and safe for long term use. They decrease both the swelling and the inflammation in the mucous membrane. *However, there are no studies showing that steroid nasal sprays or inhalers are proven to affect the Eustachian tube and decrease swelling in the middle ear.* We know that 75 percent of patients with fluid in the ear for more than three months will not clear spontaneously even at six months. [9] In these cases, the fluid will have to be drained.

Yet having said that, I will occasionally see a patient with chronic middle ear disease who has been in remission on their allergy immunotherapy suddenly get into their bad season and experience blockage of their ear. *When this occurs, often a quick dose of oral prednisone, coupled perhaps with an antihistamine, can open up their ears. But this has to be started within a week or so of when their ear blockage first occurs.* This will relieve the vacuum but not fluid once it settles in.

The obvious advantage of medication is that it is usually quick-acting. If you have sudden exposure to a friend's pet or walk into a moldy building and get congested, then immediately taking an antihistamine, if they are effective for you, is the thing to do. It will usually start to work within half an hour. Some people have a bad allergy season that lasts for a few weeks each year, and antihistamines or inhaled corticosteroids are an excellent way to manage those symptoms for several weeks or a few months. Remember, though, medications mask symptoms. As effective as they may be, they do not alter your body's underlying response to these exposures; only allergy immunotherapy can do that.

ANTI-IgE THERAPY

A new strategy to combat allergic reactions in the body is to block the effects of IgE at their very source. Many of the white cells responsible for our body's defenses against foreign substances, such as bacteria and allergens, have hundreds of sites for IgE on each cell. These IgE receptors pick up antibodies floating in your bloodstream. When the antibodies and IgE receptors unite, they trigger the inflammatory cascade we will describe in detail in the last chapter, *To Your Doctor*. Scientists have now developed an IgE-blocking antibody which effectively blocks almost all the IgE sites on the white cells, leaving no place for the antigen to bind to the cells. This is like playing musical chairs. If blocking molecules fills all the IgE receptor chairs, the allergen cannot find a seat. It loses! If it cannot bind to the receptor, no allergic reaction can occur.

The anti-IgE medication is called Xolair (omalizumab). It was initially designed to be used for patients with life-threatening asthma,[25] and its initial cost to the patient was over $30,000 a year. The cost is now down to about $1,000 per month, and it is being used for moderately severe asthmatics. It is very effective. However, its benefits only last about a month. (Like a red traffic light on a corner, once it turns green, it no longer stops the cars.) It does not truly alter the immune system and reduce your overall response the way immunotherapy does. So if you were to take anti-IgE for allergies, you would be committed to this very expensive treatment for life. Of course, the drug company is trying to get the indications for use to be extended to common allergy sufferers, but as of this writing, its use is limited to asthmatics with life-threatening disease and patients with chronic sinusitis.

For the sake of completeness, I should mention here a new device that, although not a medication, is considered a treatment. This device is designed to blow air into the nose and open the Eustachian tube so that air displaces the fluid in the middle ear. There are a few recent studies showing that the device is beneficial and effective, but there have been no long-term studies. [Previous ear inflator balloons (first described in the 1800s) have been shown to work for only a week or two at the most.] It is interesting that the federal government's own National Institutes of Health provided a grant for almost $1 million to help the drug/device company pay for testing. This study was inspired and promoted by the manufacturer, who orchestrated the clinical study and the grant application to the National Institutes of Health.

Ironically, the National Institutes of Health has consistently refused to support studies necessary to validate the effectiveness of immunotherapy for the treatment of chronic middle ear fluid — for which the international community of otolaryngologists has been calling for twenty years. Actually, Dr. George Shambaugh called for such studies beginning in 1962, and every international symposium on middle ear disease has asked for these studies to be done, to no avail. Money from pharmaceutical houses talks, but children with ear fluid aren't the only ones with a deaf ear — so is organized medicine.

OSTEOPATHIC, CHIROPRACTIC, AND ACUPUNCTURE TREATMENTS

Chiropractic

Dr. Hurst -

I have had two of my cousins tell me that they have taken their children (under a year) to a chiropractor for ear infections. Since going, their children have not had an ear infection. Do you have any history of chiropractic care for the prevention of ear infections??

Of course, there should be a word of caution here because there are many types of treatment that never have and never will prove their effectiveness for recurrent ear infections, let alone fluid. For example, there is no published evidence showing that osteopathic manipulations of the skull or chiropractic manipulation of the spine will effect a greater percent of cure than time alone. Remember that 83 percent of acute otitis cases will resolve spontaneously without any medical intervention whatsoever. How can manipulation of the cranial sutures — which are solidly fixed bones of the skull by the age of 2, be moved by your well-intentioned osteopath? Chiropractors and osteopaths can do marvels for backs and sprains, but not for otitis or chronic middle ear fluid caused by allergies.[26]

Chiropractic

Dear Dr. Hurst,

I got a little discouraged when I saw one of your replies on your web page. You told a mother to "go ahead" and have tubes put in their daughter's ear. ...You might be thinking: Chiropractic!!??? For ear infections!?!??? But they don't have back pain, they have ear infections!!!!

Don't take my word for it at face value. Check into it further. I don't know if you have a preconceived notion about chiropractic. But if you are a true man of science, I think you owe it to all of your patients to recommend all methods of care before throwing the towel into surgery. Chiropractic first, pills second, and surgery last.

Yours in Health,

Paul B, DC

Reply:

Five electronic databases were searched for all randomized clinical trials of chiropractic manipulation as a treatment of non-spinal pain. They were evaluated according to standardized criteria. RESULTS: Eight such studies were identified. They related to the following conditions: fibromyalgia, carpal tunnel syndrome, infantile colic, otitis media, dysmenorrheal and chronic pelvic pain. Their methodological quality ranged from mostly poor to excellent. Their findings do not demonstrate that chiropractic manipulation is an effective therapy for any of these conditions. "CONCLUSIONS: Only very few randomized clinical trials of chiropractic manipulation as a treatment of non-spinal conditions exist. The claim that this approach is effective for such conditions is not based on data from rigorous clinical trials." [26]

The same word of caution applies to acupuncture. There are no studies showing that it is better that watchful waiting. I have nothing bad to say if it works for you, but don't waste a lot of money for months waiting for the magic to happen.

« 10 »

IMMUNOTHERAPY

"**A**llergy shots," or *allergy immunotherapy*, is the ultimate treatment option in asthma and chronic sinusitis, and therefore, by extension, for chronic middle ear disease. It has been shown conclusively that allergy immunotherapy is the only way to downregulate the immune system so the body doesn't overreact to everyday exposures.[27] As discussed in Chapter One, allergy immunotherapy fools your body and gradually turns off the hyper reactive response at the cellular level, *so you no longer make extra IgE antibodies.*[28]

Child, 9 years

Dear Dr. Hurst,

History: 9-year-old boy with chronic OME since 6-9 months of age. The condition occurs multiple times in a year and progresses until the tympanic membrane actually ruptures!

Treatment: All of the usual. Multiple antibiotics, multiple frequencies (chronic low dose, more frequent, higher doses, etc.). Occasionally antibiotics would help, but more recently the course would be the same (i.e., rupture despite antibiotics). Tubes were placed twice. Finally, after many requests, he was referred to an allergist. The allergist diagnosed multiple allergies (dust, mold, animals, etc.) based on a skin test and prescribed an inhaler. He has started shots and no infections for 6 months!

D.B.

Furthermore, after a short duration on allergy immunotherapy you no longer release extra inflammatory cells and you no longer produce extra chemicals like histamine, so your body stops generating an allergic response. It's like gradually turning down the volume on the television: the picture may always be there, but you just don't hear the sound anymore. Your body is always able to produce an allergic response if overstimulated, but in general it stops misbehaving.

Does immunotherapy work? As mentioned earlier, immunotherapy is so effective for asthma that even *the World Health Organization says that anyone taking two or more medications for asthma should be offered immunotherapy.*[29] (The WHO has made this recommendtion since 1999 – and how many of your friends with asthma have been offered immunotherapy?) There are now several studies that show that immunotherapy even has a preventative benefit. A large study from Denmark (143 patients) showed that 45.3 percent of children with allergic nasal symptoms treated *only with medication* went on to developed asthma. The development of asthma was reduced to only 16.6 percent of an identical group of children if in addition they received immunotherapy.[4] This study is earth-shaking because it demonstrates that *allergy immunotherapy can actually prevent asthma* from developing in children who only have allergic rhinitis by almost two thirds. If it is effective for these more debilitating chronic diseases, it certainly will be effective for chronic middle ear disease.

People always ask, "How does allergy immunotherapy work?" Allergy immunotherapy actually involves injecting under the skin small doses of the substance you are allergic to. If you are allergic to dust or ragweed, we would inject you with very minute (homeopathic) amounts of the natural substance, such as a dose of dust or ragweed pollen. People naturally wonder how giving you something you are allergic to will cause your body to stop reacting. Technically, allergy immunotherapy produces blocking antibodies and causes a reduction in IgE antibody production.[28]

When talking to my patients, I often use a football team analogy to illustrate how immunotherapy works. When your immune system is overexposed to a lot of what you are allergic to, dust for example, your body produces extra dust antibodies. It is like having a hundred players out on the allergy-causing antibody team and just one little dust antigen on the other team, so every time some dust comes along, there's a massive pileup on this one little dust player. What immuno-therapy does is balance out the opposing allergy-antibody team by "shooting in" a lot of little dust players on the other team. Each allergy-antibody player is then tied up with a dust player so both sides are evenly matched. Now when an extra little "dustman" walks out onto the field, there's no one left from the antibody side to pounce on him, so he strolls down the field without producing an overreac-tion to his presence: touchdown!

Similarly, a patient with untreated allergies has a lot of extra antibodies, so when he's exposed to dust in his bedroom, the antibodies pounce on it and release a lot of histamine and he gets sick. After just a few months on immunotherapy, the antibody players are all tied up. Now when he's exposed to some dust, he's able to walk through the room and not get sick. His body has run out of unop-posed players. The real magic is that often after a short time, the antibody team gets tired; the immune system gets bored. "If no one is going to play with us, this is no fun!" So they take their IgE ball and go home. Gradually, more and more antibody players leave the field, and in a short time the shots can be extended from once a week to every other week and even further.

After four to five years of immunotherapy, the body is back to normal, and when patients can go three or four weeks between shots and be symptom-free, they can stop the shots. *They are cured of their allergy!* They usually remain free of allergy symptoms for many years, if not forever. Unless a patient has asthma in addition to chronic middle ear or sinus disease, it is my experience that they have a 90 percent chance of remaining symptom-free after a full course of immunotherapy.

Time course of biomarkers during immunotherapy

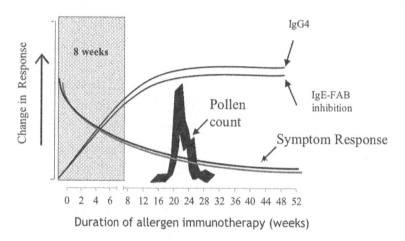

Figure 14: Effectiveness of immunotherapy.[28]

Symptoms diminish at 14 weeks as IgG4 blocking antibodies increase on immunotherapy.

Allergy immunotherapy done according to the AAOA guidelines is more than 90 percent successful for preventing further disease for patients with allergic rhinitis, and more than 85 percent successful for patients with chronic middle ear disease.[21]

I tell my patients who have chronic sinusitis that they will probably notice an improvement on allergy shots within ten to twelve weeks — they will have fewer symptoms and require less medication.

Certainly after four months on allergy therapy they should notice a significant improvement. They may not be 100 percent better, but they will know they are heading in the right direction. Patients with asthma usually notice a similarly rapid improvement, but I tell them that since the surface area of the lung is so much larger than that of the sinuses it may take six to twelve months before they're using less medication and taking fewer trips to the emergency room.

For children who come to the office with chronic middle ear fluid and significant hearing loss, the first order of business is to get their hearing back to normal. As previously discussed, this requires placing aeration tubes in the eardrum and sucking the fluid out so they can hear again. I tell their parents that once the tubes are in, the hearing will get back to normal immediately. The tubes usually stay in about a year, giving us time to test for allergies and begin treatment so their ears will not fill back up with fluid when the tubes come out.

Does this work? Throughout the world, among children who require a first set of tubes, 20 percent will need a second set put in because of recurring fluid or infection. I found in over 20 years of treating children that fewer than 4 percent needed a second set of tubes once I started allergy immunotherapy for these patients. This is five times better than the world average. It's certainly not perfect, but it's a major improvement over any other treatment modality for children with chronic middle ear fluid. Once the fluid has been removed and immunotherapy has been started, patients find within two to six months that their ears have stopped draining if they have perforations or tubes that used to drain when their allergies were acting up. They actually stop producing recurring fluid.

HOW IS IMMUNOTHERAPY ADMINISTERED?
WHAT IS INVOLVED?

After an initial evaluation and some testing, this treatment is really quite convenient. Actually, the testing itself is not so bad because with Emla® cream containing Xylocaine applied to the skin, children, and even some adults, don't feel the testing shots. After test results have identified specific allergens, patients are placed on a regimen of having one or two shots (simultaneously) every week.

Allergy shots themselves are done using a very small needle. A tiny amount of clear allergy solution (0.05 to 0.3 cc) is injected subcutaneously – just into the fatty layer under the skin. Fat has no nerve fibers so there is no pain. The only discomfort is a quick small prick in the skin. This is not like a flu shot which involves a much larger needle and a larger volume of solution injected into the muscle. After three months of gradually increasing the strength of the allergy shots patients reach a maintenance dose. At this dose most all patients can do their shots themselves at home. Only those with severe asthma must continue at the doctor's office.

But do we give shots to babies and little children? Of course not. We treat them with drops that a parent puts under their tongue. This is very effective and so safe that *all* allergists agree it can be done at home, even through the build-up phase.

If you have read and understood this little book, you are now armed with powerful information to bring your ears or your child's ears back to "normal" through the right course of testing, treatment, and follow-up with the right medical specialists. *You or your child has the right to normal hearing and a life free of debilitating allergy symptoms.* It is up to you to demand the right treatment.

Take this book to your family physician or pediatrician. Ask them to pay special attention to the last chapter, *To Your Doctor.* If they won't read it, or dismiss you by saying they don't "believe" allergies cause chronic middle ear disease, find another doctor, one who is interested in you or your child getting well.

Information is power; use it effectively for your child's sake. With a little courage and time, you can locate an ENT physician who practices allergy and understands

— yes, actually "believes" — that chronic middle ear disease is an allergic disease. They know it can be cured with immunotherapy.

Finding the right doctor to manage your allergy therapy is like marrying the right partner. The father of a friend of mine gave this sage advice when notified that his son was getting married: "If you marry the right woman, there ain't nothin' like it! If you marry the wrong woman, there ain't nothin' like it!!"

Find the *right* allergy doctor — an ear, nose, and throat surgeon who does allergy immunotherapy — and *cure* your chronic middle ear fluid. Ain't nothin' like it!

Go to AAOAF.org or PAAS.org to find an ENT allergist in your area.

Adult, 29 years

Dear Dr. Hurst,

In the past few years, I have steadily experienced more ear/sinus problems (I am a 29-year-old female). I take various OTC (over-the-counter) sinus medications (on a daily basis) for symptoms that include headaches, sinus pressure, stuffy nose, and plugged ear (usually my right ear). The headaches and sinus pressure get much worse when the weather is bad (rain or snow).

During the week, I get up at 5:00 a.m. and usually take two sinus pills (sometimes it is necessary to take more in the afternoon). This seems to keep my symptoms at bay during the week. However, on weekends I wake up several hours later. Within an hour of getting out of bed, my right ear plugs up. It usually takes several hours to half a day for it to unplug (after taking two sinus pills). Why is this happening, and what can be done about it? I'm also concerned about having to take this medication daily.

Additionally, I seem to have daily drainage...I'm constantly clearing mucus from my throat, especially after I eat a meal. I would really appreciate any advice you have for me.

Thanks, JS

Reply:

Dear JS,

You are describing the classic allergy symptoms of the whole upper respiratory tract—your nose, eustachian tubes (causing the blocked ears), and mucous in your nasopharynx (back of throat). You are lucky you do not also have asthma! Your observation that a change in the weather makes you worse strongly suggests mold allergy.

Follow the formula outlined on my web page (www. earallergy com):

1) Get a blood test, preferably the THABEST by
   MOLECULAR MEDICINE.
2) See an ENT allergist.
3) Have tubes put in to buy time to find out what
   your allergies are and get them treated.
4) Understand that allergy shots will give better
   relief without side effects, allow you to avoid
   drugs and are the only way to alter the
   immune system so you can get better and
   stay cured.

Good luck,
Dr. Hurst

« 11 »

TO YOUR DOCTOR –
THE SCIENCE

*A technical chapter for doctors and others who wish to
read further and judge the scientific evidence for themselves.*

As clinicians you understand *how* to manage a problem. When a child comes in with a case of chronic middle ear disease, sinusitis, or asthma, you know *what* to do. Your mind immediately starts thinking of the proper antibiotic or which inhaled steroid or which X-ray, etc., should be selected to treat this patient. What I would like to ask is that you step back a little and ask yourself the more basic questions, specifically:

Why is it that this patient is returning with chronic disease?

Why is it that after the first time you treated him or her for sinusitis or middle ear infection, they didn't remain free of infection?

Nicholas, age 7

Dear Dr. Hurst:

Nicholas is a 7-year-old boy who has had multiple bouts of ear infections with prolonged effusions. Beginning this spring, he has begun to cough in a staccato fashion and wheezes on exertion. His symptoms are helped a great deal by Dimetapp and Albuterol syrup. His parents have been

98

reluctant to pursue an allergic etiology for Nicholas's frequent ear infections and respiratory infections, but are now interested in determining what he might be allergic to. They live in an old house with a damp basement, one cat, and one dog.

On exam, Nicholas's nasal passages are very boggy and edematous. His ear drums are dull pasty-gray in appearance and he had stiff tympanograms today. I can detect a slight increased wheeze in the expiratory phase of respiration and his peak flow is a low 140. I have drawn the THABEST panels which you have recommended along with a total IgE. He is allergic to animals, dust, molds, and some weeds. How shall I proceed?

Sincerely,

William B. PA-C

My approach is to look *first* at the underlying physiology and mechanisms that can explain the chronic inflammation and disease a particular patient is having.

New evidence from the fields of cellular biology and immunology explain the basics of allergic reactions, how allergies can most accurately be diagnosed, and how allergy may contribute to the development of chronic inflammatory disease throughout the unified airway, including the middle ear.

You have come to know asthma as a "hyper reactive airway disease." But allergy itself is really hyper reactive *mucosal* disease. You recall that the entire upper respiratory tract — including the lungs, sinuses, Eustachian tubes, nose, and middle ear — are all lined by pseudostratified, ciliated, columnar epithelium. This mucous membrane responds similarly regardless of its location. The inflammatory process is categorized by the location, i.e., bronchitis in the lung, sinusitis in the sinuses, conjunctivitis in the eye, or otitis media in the middle ear.

As physicians, you are familiar with the fact that there are many ways to categorize a disease. Different subspecialties look at categorizing chronic sinusitis by cell type, bacteria, CAT scan findings, etc. Chronic middle ear inflammation can likewise be categorized in a number of ways. It can be categorized by the appearance of the eardrum or the thickness of the fluid, that is, is it thick "mucoid" or thin "serous" fluid. Modern immunologists throughout the world have agreed on a categorization system for sinusitis and asthma based on our knowledge of T cell activity and basic immunology.

Since we are dealing with chronic inflammation, it would be appropriate to use the same standard of classification based on immunologic findings as has been adopted in the nomenclature guidelines published by both the European and American Academies of Allergy and Clinical Immunology in 2001 and 2003 respectively.[30] They classified the inflammation found in patients with asthma or sinusitis as being either "allergic or nonallergic." I suggest that we should adopt this same system to categorize the inflammation we encounter in the middle ear. (Figure 15)

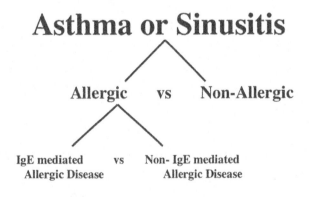

Figure 15: Classification of Allergic Disease

Under the allergic category, these academies further divided the inflammation in these target organs into "IgE or non-IgE mediated disease." This categorization system fits nicely with the concept of immunology we are about to define.

THE INFLAMMATORY CASCADE

Our current knowledge of basic response to an irritant or foreign protein is based on the difference between Thymus Type 1 and Thymus Type 2 cells. These were first discovered in mice in 1986 and referred to as Th-1 and Th-2 responses.[31] First we must determine if the patient demonstrates a nonallergic, or normal, Th-1 response, or an allergic (atopic) Th-2 response. If the response is allergic, it is further broken down into either IgE mediated or non-IgE mediated. What do we mean by this? Genetically, there are only two types of people in the world: the nonallergic, or "normal," Th-1 group and the allergic Th-2 type.

Figure 16 shows the basic distinction whereby an antigen, be it bacteria or allergen, is presented by the antigen presenting cells (APC) to a naïve T cell (Th-0 cell). There are then two pathways to choose: a Th-1 pathway or a Th-2 pathway.

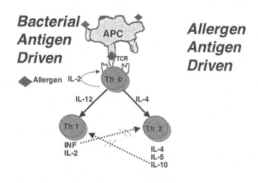

**Non-Allergic (Th 1)
 vs Allergic (Th 2)**

Figure 16: Th-0 to either Th-1 or Th-2

All normal individuals when presented during an infection by bacterial antigen stimulate a Th-1 response that is mediated by the cytokines interferon gamma (INFγ) and IL-2 (Figure 17). This produces a cellular immunity, so named because it stimulates further recruitment of macrophages and neutrophil cells in what we understand to be a classic inflammatory response to bacterial infection with rubor, dolor, calor, and tumor (redness, pain, fever, and swelling).

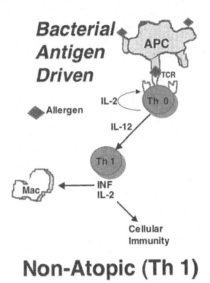

Non-Atopic (Th 1)

Figure 17: Th-1 Pathway

In response to allergen proteins, an entirely different response by the naïve Th-0 cell occurs. Allergen triggers the naïve T cell to become a Th-2 cell. This Th-2 response is mediated by an entirely different set of cytokines: IL-3, IL-4, IL-5, and IL-10 and RANTES (Figures 18, 19). IL-3 stimulates mast cells and basophiles to release IgE, tryptase, and histamine. This is a classic "IgE mediated early response" (the trapezoid in Figures 18, 19). Il-4 will also stimulate B cells that again release IgE.

102

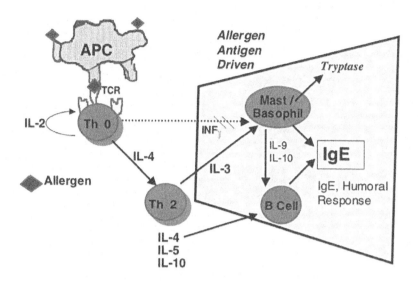

Allergic (Th 2)
early phase

Figure 18: Th-2 Pathway, Early Phase

There is also the late-phase response triggered by IL-5 and eosinophils. This non-IgE mediated delayed response (the eosinophil cells below the trapezoid boxed cells in Figure 19) is most classically seen in asthma. All these mediators have been demonstrated in the middle ear fluid and mucosa from patients with chronic middle ear disease.[10]

You are no doubt familiar with the Gell Coombs classification of inflammation. Consider the fact that this was brilliantly devised in 1973, long before there was any knowledge of inflammatory cells that we know so much about today. A classic Gell Coombs Type I response happens to be the classic IgE mediated immediate response of anaphylaxis. Gell Coombs Type II, III, and IV responses are not IgE mediated. This is understood more clearly when we look at the diagram and see that Th-2 cells also release IL-5. This cytokine

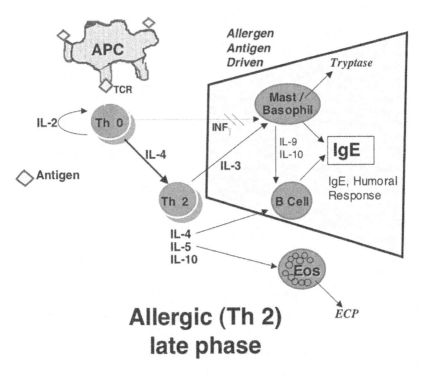

Allergic (Th 2) late phase

Figure 19: Th-2 Pathway, Late Phase

stimulates the recruitment of eosinophils (the "eos" cells below the boxed cells in Figure 19). These eosinophils are the major instigators in non-IgE mediated allergic inflammation. In medical school, we learned to do nasal smears and look for eosinophils. We were taught that this was a nonspecific sign of allergy, as was a high eosinophil count on a CBC. Yet, come to think of it, the eosinophils have nothing to do with IgE, nor the release of tryptase. That classic marker of allergy comes almost solely from mast cells. So what do eosinophils have to do with allergy?

Until 1980, allergists strongly argued that asthma had nothing to do with allergic disease because they were unable to find either tryptase or mast cells in the lung. It wasn't until after the discovery and understanding of the Th-1, Th-2 paradigm that they realized that the eosinophils are classic markers of the late-phase allergic response.

Dr. Per Venge discovered the chemical mediator released by eosinophils. He called this "eosinophilic cationic protein," or "ECP." This, with another eosinophil-derived chemical called major basic protein, or MBP, are the major mediators responsible for the inflammation that produces the late-phase response in asthmatics. These mediators are very deleterious to the upper respiratory tract mucosa, as they destroy epithelium, paralyze cilia, and recruit other inflammatory cells, including neutrophils, and more eosinophils. ECP also delays apoptosis, or cell death, so there is no normal end to the inflammation. (I had the good fortune to have Dr. Venge as my mentor and advisor during the eight years I was working on my Ph.D. dissertation.)

Take a moment to again study Figures 18 and 19. They help to demonstrate the difference between IgE mediated and non-IgE mediated allergic responses. The immediate "early" response involving mast cells, B cells, and the release of IgE is totally separate from the non-IgE mediated "late phase" response that involves the eosinophils (below the cells in the trapezoid in Figure 19). This helps explain why, as mentioned earlier, certain drugs and certain allergy tests may or may not be effective. The immediate response with mast cells causes the release of histamine. This leads to immediate sneezing, watery eyes, and a runny nose. Antihistamines may work — but only for the immediate response.

The late response, on the other hand, involves predominantly eosinophils. They have been recruited by Il-5, RANTES, and Il-4. They release ECP and major basic protein, as stated. This happens at four or more hours into an allergic response, and since no histamine is released, antihistamines do NOT reduce the symptoms. Since this was not understood until the mid-1980s, general allergists refused to acknowledge that allergy could be causing asthma — most of which is a late inflammatory phase response. Antihistamines had proven to be of little value in the treatment of asthma. This inflammatory disease is best controlled by oral or inhaled corticosteroids, which now are the mainstay of asthma management. Corticosteroids are the only medicines we have which inhibit the inflammatory effects of eosinophils and the mediators they release in the late phase of asthma, chronic sinusitis, urticaria, and allergy in general.

Why am I telling you all this? Because in order to prove a relation of allergy to asthma or sinus disease, researchers had to demonstrate tryptase from mast cells and, more importantly, ECP from eosino-phils, in the lung and sinuses. This has been done and is now accepted medical fact. But in 1988, when I did my first study on 20 patients with allergy and chronic OME, there was no evidence for tryptase or ECP in the middle ear. Thus there was no sign of mast cell or eosinophil activity in middle ear disease. That is what I had to find to prove scientifically that allergy was involved in chronic OME. And that is what I did over the next ten years.

We have successfully demonstrated tryptase in the middle ear fluid of allergic patients — and not in the ears of normal adults or children.[32, 33] Other investigators have since confirmed much of this. We have also demonstrated specific IgE in the middle ear fluid in allergic patients, and not in their serum.[34] Finally, we have demon-strated that when children or adults with longstanding chronic middle ear disease are evaluated for allergy, 100 percent of them are proven to be allergic by intradermal skin testing (the gold standard).[21] Furthermore, when these OME patients are treated for their allergies by avoiding their offending food or by allergy immunotherapy (shots), over 90 percent will resolve and remain free of middle ear fluid. An interesting side note: *There is not a single article based on good science in the world literature that remotely suggests that allergy has NO relation to chronic middle ear disease and middle ear fluid.*

In the summer of 2006, I was invited to be on a panel at an international conference attended by allergists and otolaryngologists from the European academies. My topic was "Allergic otitis: does it exist?" I contemplated that topic for some time and then it dawned on me that it was sort of like asking Christopher Columbus to talk about whether or not he thought the earth was round. To me there was no doubt about it, but how could I convince the uninformed masses — in the fifteen minutes allotted?

The fact that physicians still ask "Does allergic otitis exist?" means they really have not kept up at all with the literature, and so this is how I approached it: I discussed what we now know based on the latest studies, and I reviewed why there are lingering doubts among physicians about whether allergic otitis exists, and if there is any factual basis for those doubts.

Christopher Columbus should have known that the world was round because the Greeks in 830 BC had deduced that, since Earth was casting a shadow on the moon, it was obvious that it must be a sphere. The Greeks had worked out the diameter of the earth, as well as the seasons, and had concluded that the earth was indeed orbiting around the sun. The Arabs in 800 AD had even calculated the earth's circumference to be 24,000 miles. But all that knowledge was lost due to poor or nonexistent means of communication, and previously known truths had to be rediscovered. So it is with allergic otitis: We've had the information for many, many years, but sometimes the physicians in one country haven't stayed abreast of what others have discovered. Now with the Internet, we can review the literature from almost every medical journal in the world.

Proof of the hypothesis that chronic OME is an allergic disease requires four steps. *First*, establish a relevant, associated, objective diagnosis of atopy in patients with persistent effusion or middle ear drainage. This was done in 100 percent of both our treatment and control patients.[21] Other investigators using objective intradermal and in vitro testing have similarly demonstrated that 72 to 100 percent of children with otitis media with effusion are atopic. (See Table I at the end of this chapter.)

Second, establish an association of allergic Th-2 immune-mediated histochemical reactivity within the target organ itself. As stated earlier in this book, the middle ear is exactly like the sinuses and lung in that it is lined by pseudostratified, ciliated, columnar epithelium. This epithelium presumably must respond the same in the middle ear as it does everywhere else. Simplistically, all that has been made known about allergic inflammation of the mucosa in the nose, as regards sinusitis, and in the lung as regards asthma should be able to be extrapolated to the mucosa in the middle ear. Actually, that is just what we and others have done.

The concept that active immunologic processes may be localized phenomena in the middle ear has been established in animal models[35] as well as in humans. Lymphocytes necessary for antibody production are recruited nonspecifically into the mucosa in otitis media. T lymphocytes are common in serous or mucoid effusions.[36] The finding of CD3+ T cells has been thought to be a marker which can be used to distinguish between allergic and nonallergic sinusitis.[37] IL-5 is produced predominately by stimulated Th-2 and not by Th-1 cells[38], and is increased during the late-phase reaction of chronic middle ear disease.[39]

Proof of a relation of allergy to asthma or sinus disease required researchers to demonstrate tryptase from mast cells and, more importantly, eosinophil cationic protein (ECP) from eosinophils in the lung and sinuses. Studies in China, Japan, the US, Canada, and Sweden have demonstrated that all the mediators required for a Th-2 inflammatory response, including ECP, tryptase, and/or IL-5 mRNA cells, CD3+ T cells,[33] eosinophils,[40] mast cells,[32] RANTES,[41] prostaglandins,[42] and specific IgE for foods and inhalants[43] are present in the majority of ears with chronic effusion. Having CD3+ cells and, more importantly, cells actually manufacturing IL-5 mRNA in middle ear mucosa biopsies, provides strong evidence that the middle ear is actively participating in a Th-2 response.[33, 44]

Anti-tryptase antibody (AA1) staining has shown that mast cells are present in the mucosa and submucosa in atopics and not in controls.[32] Lasisi looked at the secretion of IgE in the middle ear of patients with chronic suppurative otitis media (CSOM) and controls. He found that "allergy appears to play a contributory role in CSOM and elevated IgE in the middle ear secretions suggests a likely mucosal response."[43] Furthermore, he found a positive skin reaction in 80 percent of CSOM, suggesting a "substantial potentiating role of allergy in SOM."

The *third step* needed to prove that the middle ear behaves as a target organ of allergy is to demonstrate that the inflammation within the middle ear is truly allergic by its nature, and not merely coincidental. That requires an examination of the epidemiology mechanisms, and treatment studies for patients with chronic otitis media with effusion.

OME is a multifacatorial disease, of which allergy is only one risk factor. Parental smoking, day-care classrooms with more than six students, asthma, and viral upper respiratory infection are also known to predispose one for OME. Yet allergy adds unique comorbidity. Allergy magnifies any of the previously named risks by a factor of 2 to 4.5 times that seen in nonallergic people.[8, 45] Thus, a child who gets an episode of acute otitis media is up to 4.5 times more likely to develop OME if that same child is also allergic.

Evidence of a direct connection comes from several controlled studies. Several of these were reviewed in Chapter Two, others are discussed shortly under "Mechanisms responsible for otitis media with effusion."

Based on skin prick testing (SPT), a Greek study[8] found a much higher incidence of allergy among 88 children with chronic OME than in the controls. They concluded that allergy is an independent risk factor for developing OME. A study in Mexico found that 15 percent of 80 children with positive skin tests to dust, corn, and cockroach had abnormal tympanograms as compared to fifty controls who all had normal Type A tympanograms, and all were SPT negative for the same three allergens. Among children with rhinitis, allergy presented an increased risk for difficulty in opening their Eustachian tubes.[46]

Doner[47] evaluated two groups of children who all had a previous M&T and adenoidectomy. Among 22 children who required repeat M&T, 36.4% had positive skin tests. This compared to a control group of 24 with *no recurrence* of their middle ear disease. Only 8 percent of these controls had positive skin tests. They concluded that allergy seemed to be a major contributing factor for recurrent disease.

Direct demonstration of serum and middle ear immunoglobulins being associated with a Th-2 response in the middle ear itself has been provided by Hamid,[42] Lasisi,[43] Sobol[44] and Hurst.[34] The evidence is conclusive enough for the 2004 guidelines published by the academies of Pediatrics, Family Practice, and Otolaryngology-Head and Neck Surgery to conclude that the middle ear epithelium of atopics has all the components required to behave in a manner similar to that of the rest of the upper respiratory system, and that "like other parts of respiratory mucosa, the mucosa lining the middle ear cleft is capable of an allergic response."[2]

The *fourth and final step* needed to prove the hypothesis of an allergy connection requires direct evidence of a dose response curve and consistency of results. A call for treatment studies has been made every four years at the International Symposium On Otitis Media, as well as by the Committee On Guidelines, which states "no recommendation is made regarding allergy management...based on insufficient evidence of therapeutic efficacy or causal relationship between allergy and OME."[2] For more than three decades, no university has taken up the challenge.

Sporadic reports of therapeutic efficacy of immunotherapy for OME have lacked documented controls until recently. In a study of 89 patients aged 4 to 70 with intractable middle ear disease, who presented with chronic effusion or chronic draining perforations or tubes, all proved to be atopic by intradermal skin testing. All were offered allergy immunotherapy based on the results of their intradermal testing. Twenty-one individuals self-selected to be "control cohorts" by choosing for a variety of reasons not to proceed with IT. Specific allergy immunotherapy completely resolved 87 percent of 127 diseased ears (an odd number because some patients had their ear disease limited to only one side). An additional 5.5 percent were significantly improved but since they still had an occasional relapse during their active allergy season such as when ragweed came out in the summer they could not be considered completely cured. All children <15 and most adults resolved within four months and remained free of disease. None of the control's ears (n=39) resolved spontaneously. (p<0.001)

The average OME patient proved to be sensitive to nine allergens (range 4–15). This study documented that in a select population, anti-allergy therapy is efficacious in preventing or limiting the duration of OME while comparing treatment patients to a control cohort.[21]

Since chronic otitis has been shown to be a low-level IgE-mediated disease similar to allergic rhinitis, with two-thirds of OME patients having a serum IgE <100 (mean 93.8μg/L);[10] intradermal testing was chosen for its greater sensitivity and reproducibility as the test for atopy. Immunotherapy was chosen to treat the underlying allergy because it has been shown to have a long-lasting effect on T lymphocytes, it acts in the earliest stages of immunologic response,

Resolution of Effusion

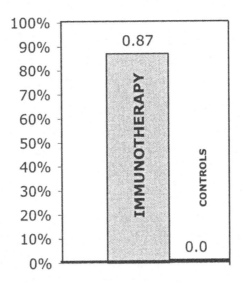

Figure 20. Resolution of patients with chronic middle ear effusion and/or drainage from their perforation or tube.[21]

and it can revert an atopic from a Th-2 response back to being a normal Th-1 responder.[27] This has been documented in cases of asthma, allergic sinusitis, and now clinically in chronic OME.[21]

This cohort study demonstrated conclusively that almost all patients with chronic middle ear fluid were atopic. Eighty-seven percent of patients who presented with draining tubes, draining perforations, or a history of OME resolved and stayed free of disease. Their follow up during the study was from one to eight years from the time of initiation of their allergy immunotherapy. They have all been followed for another 3 years and still none of these have failed, while none of the controls ever resolved spontaneously.

Direct proof that allergy contributes to chronic OME and/or other manifestations of chronic middle ear disease is best done by a randomized, DBPC trial. None have been published. It should also be noted that there has never been a study published using objective testing and controls which proves the null hypothesis.

This should not be construed to suggest that all OME is the result of allergy. What makes the middle ear mucosa the target organ of some allergies and the lung, sinuses, or skin the target of others is unknown. Having said that, just because not all allergics get otitis is no longer an excuse to ignore the role allergy plays in over 87 percent of those adults and children who present with chronic OME.

These findings are in keeping with other studies (see Table I, Appendix B) which, though lacking a control group, have also demonstrated that when patients' allergies are properly treated with IT and/or diet elimination, the effusion resolves in the majority.

MECHANISMS RESPONSIBLE FOR OTITIS MEDIA WITH EFFUSION

What about the mechanism underlying chronic OME? This too is well documented, and is generally agreed to be due to "Eustachian tube dysfunction." *But what exactly is "dysfunctional" in Eustachian tube dysfunction?* Something obstructs the Eustachian tube itself, or prevents it from opening when we swallow or yawn. The most common mechanisms that can lead to Eustachian tube dysfunction are adenoid obstruction and/or tubal edema from allergic or infectious inflammation. Fairly rarely you will encounter in your practice a patient with dystonia of the velopharyngeal muscles. As you know, these muscles extend from the Eustachian tubes and meet midline to make up the soft palate. Most all children with cleft palate have chronic OME until the cleft palate itself is repaired.

Some of these children continue to have effusion problems and require tubes on repeated occasions. In my practice, we've had two cleft palate patients whose cleft palates had been repaired, yet they continued to have persistent OME as teenagers. Their effusions resolved once allergy immunotherapy was established.

Bert, age 8

When Bert came to see me, he had already had five sets of tubes. His persistent fluid was blamed on his muscular dystrophy. It must have made his palette muscles weak, yet after treating his allergies his ears remained free of fluid for five years, after which he no longer needed allergy shots; although his dystrophy progressed such that in those 5 years he went from walking to being wheel chair bound.

Other rare causes of ET dysfunction include nasopharyngeal carcinoma, post radiation stenosis, and ciliary immotility problems associated with extremely rare congenital diseases, including Kartagene's syndrome. But these cases account for only a small fraction of the four million children (in the USA alone)[2] who develop otitis media with effusion or a draining perforation each year. Allergy and gastro esophageal reflux[15] are the best explanations for the intermittent nature of Eustachian tube dysfunction.

Bluestone[48] outlined four hypothetical mechanisms by which allergy could be responsible for Eustachian tube dysfunction leading to the production of middle ear fluid. These included: (1) the middle ear functioning directly as a "shock organ," (2) Eustachian tube dysfunction due to intrinsic mechanical obstruction from inflammatory swelling of the Eustachian tube itself, (3) inflammatory obstruction of the nose, or (4) aspiration of bacteria-laden allergic secretions from the nasopharynx into the middle ear. As hypothesized, these have all been documented to occur at times as the result of allergy.

An exhaustive review of the literature by the otolaryngology staff at the University of Pittsburgh, which sites 209 references, notes that "evidence that allergy contributes to the pathogenesis of OME is derived from epidemiologic, mechanistic, and therapeutic lines of investigation."[49] They note that "allergen-induced Eustachian tube dysfunction subverts the normal mechanisms of gas exchange into the middle ear and sets the stage for development of negative pressure and transudation of fluids into the middle ear."

Another review concurs, noting that "In patients with OME in which allergy may be a contributing factor, appropriate allergy treatment of avoidance of particular allergens, medications, and immunotherapy may be indicated."[50] Others state, "It may be prudent to screen every child with OME for allergic rhinitis and ultimately to manage those with allergic inflammation differently to nonatopic individuals with OME."[51]

Friedman[52] used a double-blind protocol to show that intranasal pollen challenge of allergic individuals produced allergic rhinitis followed by Eustachian tube obstruction. Placebo patients did not obstruct. He demonstrated twenty-five years ago that allergic reactions in the nose and nasopharynx inhibit even transient dilations of the Eustachian tube during swallowing. It should be noted that none of these patients developed effusion and middle ear fluid. This might be because of patient selection and/or the short duration of exposure. Double-blind protocols have also shown that provocative intranasal challenges with allergens or histamine produce severe functional obstruction of the Eustachian tube.[53-55]

Research into the etiology of chronic OME has provided evidence that debunks several commons myths:

We know that Eustachian tube morphology or recurrent infection does not adequately explain the pathology of otitis media with effusion, nor can adenoids acting as direct obstruction — especially in teenagers or adults who have none. Alho showed twenty years ago that "Chronic inflammation in the middle ear is a direct continuation of the acute episode in only half of the cases, and is not the result of inadequate therapy."[6] It has also been shown that "There are no substantial differences in Eustachian tube (ET) function between ears that develop OME recurrence and ears that do not."[14] Furthermore, in addition to my own papers cited earlier, review of the literature finds over a dozen studies which conclude that OME patients are indeed allergic between 74 and 100 percent of the time. Seven of these studies found that allergy management was successful in relieving the disease in 75 to 90 percent of patients. (See Table I, Appendix B.)

It is the host's immunologic response that appears to account for the differences in prognosis.

A common myth that I'm sure many patients have heard from their family physicians or pediatricians is that a child's episodes of otitis media will stop "once the Eustachian tube grows to normal size." This is simply wrong. Dr. Sade, a world-famous ear surgeon, demonstrated in 1988 that the Eustachian tubes of otitis media patients do not have "immature morphology." He performed anatomical dissections looking at the entire length of the Eustachian tube. He proved that there is no difference in size of either the isthmus or the pharyngeal portion of the ET Eustachian tube among children with chronic middle ear disease when compared with those of normal children.[13] So this chronic disease has nothing do with the size of the Eustachian tube, nor with its maturity.

Another common myth parents are told is that children prone to middle ear disease cannot equalize the pressure in their middle ears. This again is false. It was proven in 1989 by Takahashi that there is no organic obstruction or narrowing of Eustachian tube in patients with chronic middle ear disease.[56] Furthermore, Dr. Straetemans confirmed this as recently as 2005.[14] Her group measured Eustachian tube function in ears of children who develop recurrent middle ear disease and those who had no recurrence. She demonstrated that there was no substantial difference in the ability of the children in either group to be able to open or equalize the pressure in their middle ears. That is, *the Eustachian tube function in children who have recurrent disease and those who do not is the same.* Therefore, chronic middle ear disease is not because of a permanent dysfunction, nor a distortion, nor any physical abnormality of the Eustachian tube in these children. That means that something is temporarily obstructing the tube to make it not function following an illness, including a middle ear infection, a respiratory tract infection, or a cold — or an allergy attack.

A brilliant study by Hardy[57] described a new rat model in which the middle ear becomes an actual target organ for allergy. He demonstrated that exposure to transtympanic allergen induced both Eustachian tube dysfunction and formation of middle ear effusion.

What other evidence do we have of a "united airway," that is, that the middle ear, including the Eustachian tube, nose, and lung function as a unified respiratory organ? Braunstahl[58] did a brilliant study where he took nonasthmatic children who had allergic rhinitis and did nasal provocation with pollen. He then measured by bronchial washings the inflammatory cells in the lungs of these nonasthmatics and found that the nasal provocation stimulated the lung to also produce an allergic inflammatory response with increased eosinophils, etc. He concluded *that the upper respiratory tract responded as one unified airway.*

Similarly, Hamid looked at the cells in the middle ear fluid and took biopsies of middle ear mucosa, and at the same time did biopsies of the nasal pharynx mucosa just next to the Eustachian tube orifice.[42] He discovered that the inflammatory profile of middle ear effusion correlated with that in the nasal pharynx, or upper airway, and stated that allergic inflammation in atopic patients with OME occurs on both sides of the Eustachian tube. That is, he measured eosinophils, CD3 T cells, Il-4, and messenger RNA for Il-5 and found them all to be elevated in both locations. He concluded that the middle ear may behave in a "similar manner to the lungs under allergic inflammatory insults" and that the *"middle ear may be included in the united airways."* Peterson's review in *Allergy 2002*, particularly made the point that there is a weak inflammatory infiltration present in the mucosa *even in the absence of symptoms* when sub-threshold exposure to an allergen persists.[50] This is exactly the hyper reactive mucosal response that other immunologists and I use to define allergic inflammation. Hamid further states that this minimal persistent inflammation is present in mite and pollen allergy, and reiterates that it involves ICAM-1, a major receptor for human rhinoviruses.[42]

Ohashi[59] published an interesting paper showing that viral infections in children stimulated ICAM, an inflammatory precursor and attractant of eosinophils and neutrophils. This response to virus occurred only in allergic children. Viral URI in normal children did not have the same effect. Thus the scientific correlation supports what we observe when our atopic children get a URI. The virus triggers the persistent subclinical inflammation, which is constantly present in the mucosa of allergic children, to boil over into an asthmatic attack, sinus infection, or exacerbation of their middle ear disease. Nonallergic children simply never respond this way. They rarely develop chronic disease of the sinuses, lungs, or middle ear.

I should interrupt here and apologize — you probably noted that many of these references are years old. That is part of my point. This is old news but still not accepted, let alone adopted, as standard practice by most physicians. I cannot explain why this is the case.

Ebmeyer demonstrated that combined exposure to allergens and bacteria in already sensitized (atopic) animals leads to chronic middle ear disease with significantly delayed recovery compared with non-sensitized (non-atopic) mice.[60] You, of course, know this to be true. You instruct the mothers of your pediatric patients with asthma to be very careful when they develop a viral cold. You caution them to increase their children's asthma medicines and employ nebulizer machines at the earliest sign of a viral infection.

You do not have to give such warning to your nonasthmatic children when they get a viral URI, because they rarely develop asthma as a consequence. Perhaps you did not consider the underlying pathophysiology behind your instructions, but this is what is happening: Since 80 percent of your asthmatics are allergic, they are simply more vulnerable to developing more severe, long-lasting responses to a viral cold than nonallergic children — be it an asthma attack, or a chronic sinus infection, or chronic middle ear fluid. Their respiratory mucosa is hyper reactive to a viral trigger and so a viral upper respiratory infection may well precipitate an asthma attack. Hyper reactivity in this case can be compared with boiling an egg. Normal cells are like a pot of water at room temperature — drop in an egg (representing a virus infection) and nothing happens. But if the pot of water is almost ready to boil — very hot but not quite bubbling (superheated, as they say) — drop in an egg and the water instantly boils over. The mucous membrane of allergic individuals is hyper reactive in exactly the same sense.

Dr. Kakizaki's group in Japan[61] looked at 15 patients who had asthma and chronic middle ear disease vs. fifteen asthmatics with no middle ear disease. They showed that the mediator IL-5 that is essential for a Th-2 allergic response, and responsible for the accumulation of eosinophils triggering the same kind of allergic response we see in the lungs of asthmatics, is also present in the ears of children with chronic OME. This inflammatory mediator was not present in the ear mucosa of the controls. They concluded, therefore, that the IL-5 responsible for the eosinophil inflammation in these middle ears is *produced locally in the ear itself.* This suggests that the allergic reaction actually occurs in the middle ear, and again supports the idea that the middle ear is itself capable of an allergic response. Kakizaki's work supports allergy functioning as a CAUSATION of middle ear disease, not merely a correlation factor. The great unknown is why in different allergic patients the target organ is just the skin or just the sinuses or just the lungs or the ears.

Dr. Sminova and her colleagues have demonstrated that the cytokines present in middle ears play a key role as molecular regulators of middle ear inflammation.[62] In a very complicated paper, she explains in detail the immunologic mechanisms wherein cytokines can switch the acute phase of inflammation to the chronic stage and induce molecular and pathologic processes leading to the histologic changes demonstrated in ears with chronic fluid. This work is extremely important. As complex as her presentation is, it explains the immunologic basis for why some ears, following an acute episode, can change seemingly spontaneously into developing chronic effusion.

Our own paper in 2002 explained how the high level of neutrophils — usually associated with bacterial infection — present in the effusion of atopic patients can be explained when the effusion itself is sterile.[11] Infection itself can indeed be a stimulus. However, again referring to Rosenfeld's work, only 17 percent of children with acute episodes go on to develop chronic middle ear effusion.[9] (Figure 1) Now you know what is different about this select 17 percent: all are atopic.[21]

Another reason many doctors believe that allergy has nothing to do with middle ear disease is because most middle ear disease occurs in the winter months, and they simply think allergy is caused only by spring or summer pollens.[63] When I looked at which allergens were positive in my 2008 study, I found that these patients had perennial allergies. All seasons were involved. Most particularly: 95 percent of patients were allergic to dust, 62 percent to grass, and molds were positive in 88 percent of patients. This also demonstrated the failure of prick testing. Most allergists agree that a prick test equals a class 4 or more dilute test on an intradermal test scale. If that were true, prick testing would only have diagnosed 10 percent of these patients as being allergic.

DIFFERENT TESTING METHODS

Like everything else in medicine, if you *do not* use accurate and sensitive means of analysis, you *will not* successfully diagnose a significant portion of your patients. It's like the difference between getting a standard sinus X-ray (equals prick testing) vs. using a CAT scan (intradermal testing). Which would you order if you suspected chronic sinusitis? After all, the accuracy of a diagnosis is dependent on the testing methodology. I mentioned earlier, in Chapter Seven on testing, that as physicians you have had allergy patients who you were absolutely convinced had allergy, yet when you did prick testing or drew a standard RAST test, results were negative. In these cases there is a *disconnect between your clinical judgment and the lab test results.* Yet somehow we doctors tend to rely more heavily on the test results than on our own understanding of the patient's disease.

If you are a doctor in the situation where you strongly believe a patient is allergic, yet the tests you did were negative, stop and think for a minute: for a RAST test to work, you have to have a lot of specific IgE for dust, cat, or grass in order for the test to be positive. A positive test is 100 percent specific, but a negative test does not guarantee that the patient is *not* allergic or atopic. Similarly, prick testing, though highly specific, has a 50 percent false negative rate and is no better than a coin toss in diagnosing allergy. On the other hand, intradermal skin testing has the highest specificity and sensitivity with the lowest false positive rate of all testing techniques we can offer our patients.

To help understand how measuring specific IgE by RAST sometimes works and sometimes does not, let us review a little blood chemistry. If you draw a line around the room you are sitting in and that line represents all the immunoglobulins in your system, almost 76 percent, represents IgG, another 20 percent represents the IgA in your system, another 4 percent is the IgM and IgD — which leaves less than 0.002 percent of that line around the room for total IgE. When S. G. O. Johannson and Nobel prizewinner Dr. Izikawa discovered total IgE in 1986, it was a major breakthrough. They found that asthmatic patients in particular had very high levels of IgE.

Arbitrarily, it was decided that anyone with a total IgE level over 100µg was considered to be abnormal and levels below 100µg were considered "normal." Yet when the test for total IgE first came out, it was not as sensitive an assay as we have now.

RAST/ImmunoCAP were designed to be as close in sensitivity as prick testing. In many cases this is true, as a positive RAST strongly suggests allergy — but the opposite is not true. Studies show very poor correlation overall between intradermal skin testing and RAST.[64] As mentioned in the chapter on testing, *I find the THABEST micro Eliza assay to be the only reliable in vitro test.*[20]

Asthma, as it turns out, is a "high-level IgE mediated disease." Most asthmatics do indeed have levels ranging from 100µg/L to 6,000µg/L. Allergic rhinitis and certainly otitis are diseases of low IgE levels. We demonstrated with 98 chronic OME patients that their median total IgE was about 38µg/L.[10] Two-thirds of OME patients had IgE levels below 100µg/L. That helps explain Bernstein's mistaken idea — which is so often quoted — that less than one-fourth of chronic OME patients are allergic. Bernstein's 1981 study, though sentinel in being among the first to link allergy to otitis, underesti-mated the role of allergy in OME because of his very narrow definition of allergy which required both rhinitis *and* a total IgE greater than 100µg/L or positive results of prick testing,[65] This of course is not a standard definition for allergy, but explains why, *by his definition*, he only labeled 22 percent of patients with middle ear fluid as allergic. He missed the other 78 percent who had a total IgE below 100 and no rhinitis accompanying their chronic OME or those whose prick testing was negative. His error thirty years ago has become another myth leading most physicians to still believe that only 22 percent of OME patients are allergic. This has unfortunately stuck in the minds of your fellow physicians because they have not kept up with the more recent science published.

Earlier I presented to you the four steps needed to prove that allergy is responsible for chronic middle ear disease and fluid, but is there *adequate proof?* Several authors have done extensive reviews of the literature.[51] A recent (2006) and in-depth review by Tewfik concluded that the relation between allergy and OME, as strong and convincing as it is, "will remain controversial until well controlled clinical studies are conducted documenting that in select populations anti-allergy therapy is efficacious in preventing or limiting the duration of OME."[51]

At the beginning of this book, I described a crude study I did in 1988 wherein I looked at 20 patients who had already required at least three sets of aeration tubes. We showed that all these patients were atopic, and that 100 percent of those who stayed on immunotherapy remained free of disease for three years, while 100 percent of those who either refused or could not maintain their allergy treatment suffered recurrence.[1] Since that paper was published, it has been referred to in many reviews — but always with the caveat that there was no control group. I therefore designed and presented a prospective cohort study to look more carefully at the same problem. The pilot study of 39 patients was presented at the European Society of Pediatric Otolaryngology, as well as at the American Academy of Otolaryngic (ENT) Allergy in 2006. The results in an even larger number of patients (98) were published in 2008.[21] I alluded to this earlier, but it is worth reviewing in greater detail.

I began by recognizing that there are two possible explanations for the increased incidence of allergy which has been documented among patients with OME: either 1) OME is a disease merely *associated with* atopy, or, perhaps, 2) OME is *due to a true allergic response* in which the middle ear, like the nose and lung, participates directly in a Th-2 mediated allergic reaction. In that case, patients should benefit from allergy immunotherapy.

The clinical study I designed focused on patients in my private practice whose allergic status was determined using intradermal skin testing. The efficacy of allergy immunotherapy as a way to maintain these patients free of chronic middle ear fluid or drainage was considered successful if they remained clear for at least two years.

Skin prick testing was not used because of its poor reproducibility, poor specificity, and the fact that it is not quantitative. Dr. Johansson (co-discoverer of IgE) advises that *"the best correlation with RAST is obtained with a skin test that measures quantitatively the immunologic sensitization, namely a skin titration procedure where one determines the least amount of allergen giving a significant positive skin test."*[66] We therefore chose intradermal testing. Specific immunotherapy was selected as the treatment method because it acts in the early stage of immunologic response; it affects the Th-1/Th-2 ratio, is a biologic response modifier, and has long-lasting effect on T lymphocytes.[4]

Over the course of eight years, 89 patients fit the criteria for the study. Sixty-eight patients maintained their allergy immunotherapy and/or food-elimination diet for over a year. Another 21 patients, although enrolled in the study and completing their allergy testing, never maintained their therapy for one reason or another. Some patients simply refused to undergo immunotherapy; others began therapy but either moved or lost their insurance; and some simply did not believe the allergy shots would be efficacious. Some patients actually stopped therapy or moved and then returned to the practice within a year or so, but because they had not completed a full year of therapy, they were considered a cohort of control patients.

Table II, in Appendix B, shows that their mean ages were similar. The treatment group had 2.8 tubes per patient and the control group had 2.5. These were statistically identical. Both groups similarly had the same number of repeat placement of tubes, as the graph indicates. Both groups had the same ratio of male to female, and in both groups more than 30 percent had had tonsils and/or adenoids removed before being enrolled in the study. Statistically, this suggests that both groups were essentially identical and there was no apparent bias in the selection of patients for one group or the other.

The number of patients who, in addition to the chronic middle ear fluid, also presented with asthma, rhinitis, adenoidectomy and/or tonsillectomy was statistically similar. Thirteen percent presented with only unilateral disease. What is most significant is that 37 percent of the treatment group and 48 percent of the control group presented with chronic middle ear fluid or drainage *as their only symptom*. Chronic middle ear disease may often be the sole presenting symptom of allergy.

Table III, also in Appendix B, looks at both the treatment group and the control group, and shows what percentage had chronic draining tubes, retraction and/or atelectasis of the eardrums, etc. What is most important to note is that 100 percent of both the treatment group and the control group were atopic. We then looked at the efficacy of immunotherapy. As you can see from this chart, 127 involved ears of 68 treated patients resolved. This was a success rate of 91.2 percent. Yet all the control patients failed. A truly significant difference of $p<0.001$. Remarkably, 85 percent resolved completely while an additional 5.5 percent were reduced to having only one or two exacerbations during their treatment years. All the children under 15 years old were cured.

In conclusion, this cohort study of 68 patients undergoing treatment as compared to 21 control patients demonstrated conclusively that *almost all patients with chronic middle ear fluid are atopic*. It was also demonstrated that these patients rarely resolve spontaneously. More than 90 percent of patients with chronic middle ear fluid who present with draining tubes, draining perforations, or draining mastoid cavities will resolve and stay free of disease from one to five years on allergy immunotherapy.(See Figure 20, page 112.)

CHRONIC OTITIS MEDIA WITH EFFUSION IS IRREFUTABLY AN ALLERGIC DISEASE

Physicians must continually keep in mind that, in cases of chronic sinusitis and otitis media, for each individual case of "infection," the particular organism is of utmost importance. Yet the bacteriology tells us nothing about the underlying pathophysiology of the disease itself. The various bacteria, viruses, prions, and perhaps biofilms are merely opportunists. Many of these have been shown to be present but inactive in normal middle ears, which are no more sterile than is the nose. It is the host's immunologic status, i.e., whether or not they are atopic or normal, that holds the key to understanding the underlying mucosal response causing his or her sinusitis, asthma, or middle ear disease. Simply put: We all walk around with bacteria in our noses, but we are not sick. It takes the coming together of several factors under exactly the proper circumstances in a weakened host with a genetic predisposition for allergies for us to become *chronically* infected. All of us can get an infection but it is the allergic children who are more easily inoculated and have a more difficult time resolving infections. They have hyper reactive mucosa lining their entire respiratory tract — an infection waiting to happen.

In summary: Current medical evidence supports the link between allergy and OME. Application of newly gained knowledge of inflammation provided by modern immunology and cellular biology as regards other chronic mucosal inflammatory diseases of the unified airway helps clarify our understanding of the pathophysiology underlying chronic middle ear disease.

Histologic, epidemiologic, and clinical studies based on objective allergy testing have thus:
1) established, using intradermal testing, that patients with OME are almost universally atopic (Tables I, II);
2) demonstrated that all the mediators necessary for a Th-2 allergic response are present in the middle ear;
3) provided medical evidence to support the conclusion that "the middle ear (mucosa) is capable of an allergic response"[2]; and
4) shown that chronic middle ear disease does resolve with immunotherapy in over 85 percent of cases as compared to 0 percent of a control cohort.[21]

Review of recent medical evidence supports the hypothesis that chronic otitis media with effusion is an allergic disease. It raises a call for further studies to confirm that treatment using immunotherapy, an established, conventional modality recognized to be effective in treating and reversing allergic rhinitis and asthma, is worth considering for those patients with this type of otherwise seemingly intractable middle ear disease.

Thus it has been proven that:

- The middle ear, as part of the unified airway, can be a target organ of allergy.
- OME is frequently an IgE mediated, late phase, allergic disease.
- Allergy can cause Eustachian tube dysfunction.
- Skin prick testing will underestimate the incidence of allergy among patients with chronic middle ear fluid.
- Once the patient is identified as being allergic, aggressive treatment of his/her allergies with immunotherapy can frequently resolve the underlying middle ear disease.

Child, age 16 months

Dear Dr. Hurst,
After reading the information on your web site (earallergy.com), and several of your recent scientific publications, I can't tell you how strongly I agree with your conclusions. More importantly, as the parent of a 16-

month-old boy with chronic OME even following tympanostomy (ear tubes), I am relieved to see someone who agrees with my wife and me. To be honest, we knew that our son was allergic to milk, but did not realize that dairy products could be contributing to his OME. We removed all milk products from his diet.

We have seen no effusion since, the longest stretch since the tubes were put in back in November. Several of my son's MDs (we've gone to four different ENTs) have scoffed at the notion that his allergies could be contributing to his ear infections. One ENT even went so far as to tell us that he didn't believe that children under 5 could have allergies. Even the allergist wasn't convinced that food allergies could contribute to the OME.

To be honest, about a year ago, a woman in a restaurant struck up a conversation with us and told us to figure out his food allergy to eliminate his chronic ear infections (her son was allergic to corn). If only I knew then what I know now.

Anyway, I just wanted to let you know, as both a scientist and a parent, that I am very grateful for the work you are doing. I plan on bringing copies of your papers to both his pediatrician and his ENT.

Thanks again,
Brian D., Ph.D.
Laboratory of Clinical and
Experimental Endocrinology
and Immunology

It is hoped that the data in this chapter provides significantly adequate "evidence-based medicine" so that you understand and feel comfortable in agreeing with me that refractory, non-acute OME is a sign of allergic hyper reactive mucosal disease. As such, it is most effectively treated by aggressive allergy immunotherapy. It seems that it is now time to reconfigure our treatment paradigm for children and adults with chronic middle ear fluid who have been suffering with hearing loss or draining ears for years. When our standard regimen of antibiotics and tubes fails to provide more than temporary relief of our patients' propensity to re-accumulate fluid in their middle ears, we are obligated to offer them allergy testing and treatment.

Our goal should be that these patients in particular should be drug-free and symptom-free.

GOAL:

Patients should be
**DRUG FREE and
SYMPTOM FREE**

« 12 »

SUMMARY:
HOW I WOULD MANAGE A PATIENT

Patients with chronic middle ear fluid have a right to expect more from the medical community than their current experience. They should expect to have normal ears. If they have read this book and then asked you to read this chapter, they already understand that the most important question to ask you as their family physician or pediatrician is: "Why do my ears keep filling up with fluid?" Or, if they have a perforation or tubes, they have every right to ask, "Why do my ears keep getting infections and draining? Weren't the tubes supposed to stop that?" If you can't answer the "whys," you need to learn more about the problem.

The answer to these questions is quite simply that, *due to allergy,* the mucous membrane which lines the middle ear is making too much mucus, which either fills the closed middle ear space, producing chronic fluid and hearing loss, or, if there's an opening such as a perforation or tube in place, their allergy causes them to produce a lot of mucus that drains through the hole or tube. *Allergies are just about the only cause for the mucous membrane to become congested and produce more mucus.*

If your patient's nose is running clear, watery mucus all the time, and they are going through boxes of tissues, you would correctly guess that this is caused by allergies. Doctors will sometimes say, "Oh, it's 'Eustachian tube dysfunction,'" but what is it that's dysfunctional about the Eustachian tube? Quite simply, it's swollen and making too much mucus. What is really "dysfunctional" is that most physicians won't think about the underlying pathophysiology or cause of this disease process. Instead they jump on the bandwagons driven by the pharmaceutical companies — the antibiotic bandwagon and the put-in-tubes bandwagon — but very few are on an allergy bandwagon.

Now that you understand that allergies can cause this disease and you also know how best to test for allergies, what can we really do about it? Antihistamines and nasal corticosteroids don't address middle ear problems at all, although they are effective in many patients with allergic sinus or nasal symptoms. The only truly effective treatment for chronic middle ear disease is immunotherapy — allergy shots.

This is unfortunate in that it involves some testing and a three- or five-year commitment to the immunotherapy. But fortunately it works. We've demonstrated now in almost a hundred patients with chronic middle ear fluid that immunotherapy will completely cure over 85 percent of them. We've also shown through a parallel control group of patients with the exact same disease that 100 percent of those who refuse treatment continue to have fluid in their ears or persistently draining tubes for years. Not a single patient from age 4 to 50 failed to respond to treatment. All of our failures were over age 50, reflecting the scarring that results from protracted, untreated disease which sometimes simply becomes irreversible — and reason not to delay in seeking immunotherapy for your chronic middle ear disease patients.

Children you should suspect of having allergy are:

1. the child whose fluid persists for over 2 months;

2. the child who has tubes which continually drain;

3. the child with a hole in his eardrum which drains; and/or

4. the child who has failed his/her school hearing test and has no history of ear infections.

MY "3 M" PLAN

Your patients' choices are simply these three:

1. continue to be *miserable*;

2. *mask* the symptoms of middle ear congestion and fluid with temporary measures such as decongestants and even steroids; or

3. cure the problem once and for all by *modulating* their immune system with allergy immunotherapy. This is the only way to stop the body from overreacting to common environmental triggers such as dust, pollen, animals, and molds.

Do not misunderstand me: I'm not against placing tubes in the ears to treat the symptoms of congestion and hearing loss. In fact, it is absolutely essential to get the hearing back up to normal as soon as possible, because we know this fluid will not resolve spontaneously for at least six months, and then in only one quarter of patients.[9] I've seen many patients who have chosen not to put tubes in. In these patients the fluid will remain for three or four years, with varying degrees of hearing loss. I personally feel that refusal to place tubes in these cases is a type of child abuse bordering on medical negligence — be that refusal by the physician in denying appropriate referral or by a parent who is understandably anxious about the risks of anesthesia to their child.

In the case of children, this can be an absolute disaster because they are kept behind in school. Sometimes they are labeled as having learning disabilities based on hearing loss and the resulting poor performance. I've even seen this hearing loss drive some youngsters to drop out of school and one 15-year-old even attempted suicide. (Allergy therapy stopped her ears from ten years of drainage, returned her to normal hearing, and she has since gone on to college.) We also know that if you delay putting tubes in, the eardrum can be scarred and cause permanent changes in the middle ear. So I tell my parents of school children to *first get the tubes in* so as to get the hearing back to normal. This will buy a year in which to find out exactly what the allergies are *and then get the allergies under control with immunotherapy* before the tubes fall out. (Children under 12 years of age may also need their adenoids removed.)

The other important message is that once you've decided to refer your patient for an allergy evaluation, it must be with an ENT surgeon who also does allergy work. These physicians will be certified members of the American Academy of Otolaryngic Allergy (AAOA) or the Pan American Allergy Society(PAAS). In contrast, as mentioned earlier in this text, the *general* allergist is either a pediatrician or internist who has less expertise or even interest in diagnosing middle ear disease. Furthermore, because they are immunologists first, they are inundated with patients with severe asthma and AIDS, and simply seem not to want to be bothered with the seemingly minor problem of ear fluid.

General allergists test with very weak-strength solutions, so they miss more than half the allergies that are present. Their testing limits them to treat only the few things their patients are severely allergic to. Their reliance on RAST or prick testing means they cannot pick up everything. Obviously, if half of a patient's allergens go unrecognized, and therefore untreated, there is less chance of a cure. They also seem to be afraid of their own immunotherapy techniques perhaps because they have as much as a 5 percent reaction rate, including some deaths every few years, whereas the ENT allergists' reaction rate is less than half a percent — with no reported deaths. In fact, allergy shots from an ENT allergist have proved to be 30 times safer than taking a penicillin pill.[19] This safety results from the fact that the *initial treatment dose is based on a dose response curve (Figure 10)* and not on a single point from a single prick test. Even when they do diagnose allergies, they still treat their allergic asthma and sinus patients 70 to 80 percent of the time only with medication and do not offer immunotherapy. They are just masking the symptoms.

General allergists are also so concerned about allergy reactions that they never allow patients to do their shots at home, while ENT allergists in general have almost all their patients doing their maintenance immunotherapy shots at home, unless they also have significant asthma.

And what about treatment for young tots? Sublingual therapy, drops given under the tongue, is effective and especially safe. I always use these allergy drops to treat children under five. It is safe and approved for home use by all allergy academies.

What is really most important to you is to refer your patients to a specialist who's interested and capable of providing adequate immunotherapy so that their ear disease resolves. It must end, and it can with proper care.

FREEDOM !!

Patients have every right to expect a life free of chronic middle ear fluid. This disease is simply a manifestation of allergy attacking the middle ear instead of the nose, lungs, or skin. Because it is a closed space, the fluid in the ear has nowhere to run out, and for whatever reason, the usual therapies for allergic hay fever and springtime allergies are almost totally ineffective in the middle ear. The only effective option is to get adequate allergy evaluation and immunotherapy. The longer proper treatment is delayed, the longer it will be before your patient is cured.

I welcome your comments, questions or suggestions. Please contact me via my Web site or through my publisher.

Four million children with preventable and treatable
learning disabilities is a disgrace to our profession as healers.
Let's do something about it.

APPENDIX A

SPECIAL DIETS

MOLD ELIMINATION DIET

DO NOT EAT THE FOLLOWING:

Instructions: First, take this list, put it on the refrigerator and IGNORE IT!! Get a sense of what you eat that is ON the list – you are just going to STOP eating that in a week. Also get a sense of what you eat that is NOT ON the list – and you are just going to shift to eating more of what you are already used to.

*Cheese of all kinds, including cottage cheese.

*Mushrooms

*Vinegar and vinegar containing foods, such as mayonnaise and other salad dressings, catsup, chili sauce, pickled beets, relishes, green olives and mustard.

*Sour cream, sour milk, buttermilk and flavored yogurt

*Alcoholic liquors, especially beer and wine

*Soured breads, such as pumpernickel, coffee cakes and other foods made with large amounts of yeast, especially heavy yeast donuts and cinnamon buns.

*Sauerkraut

*Apple cider and home-made root beer.

*Pickled and smoked meats and fish, including delicatessen food, sausages, frankfurters, corned beef, pickled tongue, ham and bacon. (These do not contain mold, but have lots of chemicals used to "smoke" the meat. Moldy patients are often chemically sensitive also.)

*All dried fruits such as apricots, dates, prunes, figs and raisins.

*Canned tomatoes unless home-made. All canned juices. (There is nothing wrong with canned tomatoes if home made, but store bought tomato sauce and catsup are made from bruised tomatoes that have started to mold, and have added vinegar.)

*Eat only freshly opened canned foods and freshly prepared fruits.

*Do not eat meat or fish more that 24 hours old. Avoid foods if made from leftovers such as meat-loaf, hash and croquettes. Avoid hamburgers unless made from freshly ground meat. It is better to freeze leftovers if not going to be eaten in 24 hours.

*Sugar – it feeds the Candida mold normally found in your GI tract.

WARNING: DO NOT BE SURPRISED IF YOU EXPERIENCE CONTIN-UED OR INCREASED SYMPTOMS DURING THE FIRST WEEK TO TEN DAYS ON THE MOLD ELIMINATION DIET. THIS IS A RELA-TIVELY COMMON HAPPENING DURING THE INITIAL WITH-DRAWAL PHASE.

THE CANDIDA CONTROL DIET
FOODS YOU CAN EAT:

VEGETABLES
  (FRESH)
*Asparagus
*Beans
*Beets
*Broccoli
*Brussels sprouts
*Cabbage
*Cauliflower
*Celery
*Corn
*Cucumbers
*Eggplant
*Green peppers
*Greens:
  -turnip
  -spinach
  -mustard
  -beet
  -collard
  -kale
*Legumes
*Lettuce
*Okra
*Onions
*Parsley
*Parsnips
*Peas
*Radishes
*Summer and
  winter squash
  -acorn
  -butternut
  -zucchini
*Sweet potatoes
*Tomatoes
*White potatoes

FRUITS (FRESH)
*Apples
*Apricots
*Avocados
*Bananas
*Blackberries
*Blueberries
*Cherries
*Grapefruit
*Grapes
*Mangoes
*Nectarines
*Papaya
*Peaches
*Pears
*Pineapple
*Plums
*Raspberries
*Strawberries

MEATS
*Beef
*Chicken
*Clams
*Cornish hen
*Duck
*Eggs
*Goose, pheasant,
  other game birds
*Lamb
*Lobster
*Shrimp
*Pork
*Quail
*Rabbit
*Salmon and
  other fresh fish
*Tuna
*Veal

NUTS, SEEDS & OILS
  (UNPROCESSED)
*Almonds
*Brazil nuts
*Butter
*Cashews
*Filberts
*Oils (cold pressed)
  -almond
  -apricot
  -avocado
  -corn
  -linseed
  -olive
  -safflower
  -sesame
  -sunflower
*Pecans
*Pumpkin seeds

CEREAL GRAINS
*Barley
*Corn
*Millet
*Oats
*Rice
*Wheat

BEVERAGES
*Milk
*Water

*

ESSENTIALLY ANY
FRESH VEGETABLE,
FRUIT OR MEAT
IS SAFE

APPENDIX B

TABLES I, II AND III

Table I:
Studies of OME Patients with Allergy
Confirmed by Skin Testing

YEAR	AUTHOR	# PTS	% of Posi-tive Tests	% Improved with allergy therapy
'42	Dohlman[67]	178	56%	
'42	Mao[68]	252	29%	of pathologically deaf children
			2%	of normal children
'49	Jordan[69]	123	74%	98%
'58	Solow[70]	50	72%	
'61	Lecks[71]	82	88%	
'65	Fernandez[72]	113	55%	95%
'65	Whitcomb[73]	38	100%	87%
'67	Draper[74]	340	53%	91%
'81	Hall[75]	92	100%	82%
'81	McMahan[76*]	119	93%	86%
'86	Sanz[77*]	20	30%	
'88	Tomonaga[78]	259	72%	of OME cases
'90	Hurst[1++]	20	100%	100%
'91	Becker[79]	35	34%	SPT
'94	Nsouli[12*]	104	78%	86%
'94	Corey[80*]	89	61%	
'96	Hurst[23]	73	87%	
'98	Psifidis[81]	148	59%	78%
'04	Doner[47]	22	38%	SPT
'08	Lasisi[82]	80	80%	SPT
'08	Hurst[21++]	89	100%	89% resolve
				0% of controls

PTS = number of patients
++ = patients not included in previous study
* = in vitro testing SPT = skin prick test

Table II:

Demographics of Treatment and Control Cohorts

		Treatment	Control	Total	P value
# of patients		68	21	89	
Atopic - # (%)		68 (100)	21 (100)	89 (100)	ns
Sex	Male	34 (50.0)	11 (52.4)		ns
# (%)	Female	34 (50.0)	10 (47.6)		ns
Age in years	4 – 15	37 (54.4)	15 (71.4)	52 (58.4)	0.19 = ns
# (%)	16 – 51	18 (26.4)	5 (23.8)	23 (25.8)	0.85 = ns
	51 – 70	13 (19.1)	1 (4.7)	14 (15.8)	
Mean age	of Children 4-15	9.3	8.5		ns
	of all Patients	26.6	18.7		
Number of sets	No tube	11	1	12 (13.4)	
of tubes per	1 tube	19	4	23 (25.8)	
patient including	2 tubes	15	9	24 (26.9)	
those inserted	3 tubes	11	4	15 (16.8)	
during the study	4 tubes	8	1	9 (10.1)	
	5-10 tubes	3	2	5 (5.6)	
Mean # tubes / patient		1.94	2.29		0.3 = ns
Total # patients with tubes		57 (83.8)	18 (85.7)	75 (84.2)	ns
Surgical interventions	Adenoidectomy	16 (23.5)	5 (23.8)	21 (23.6)	
	or T&A	9 (13.2)	3 (14.2)	12 (13.4)	
	Total T&A + A	25 (36.8)	8 (38.0)	33 (37.0)	0.3 = ns
Mean # + allergens	by IDT	10.16	13		

Number (%)
T&A = tonsillectomy and adenoidectomy
A = adenoidectomy
P = Mann Whitney p value

Table III:

Response of 68 Patients to Immunotherapy vs. 21 Controls, from Presentation to Completion of Immunotherapy

Treatment Group	Patient Age	# Patients	% Complete Resolution	Partial Resolution	Failed
	4 – 15	37	92.2	7.8	0
	16 – 50	18	83.3	13.3	4.1
	51 - 70	13	46.2		53.8
Total		68	80.9	7.4	11.8
Controls	4 – 59	21	0	0	100

Table I, adapted from: Hurst DS: The middle ear: The inflammatory response in children with otitis media with effusion and the impact of atopy. Clinical and histochemical studies., in Comprehensive Summaries of Uppsala Dissertations from the Faculty of Medicine, Dept of Immunology and Clinical Chemistry #978. Uppsala, Sweden: Uppsala University, Sweden, 2000, p 14, with permission.

Tables II and III, reprinted from: Hurst DS. Efficacy of allergy immunotherapy as a treatment for patients with chronic otitis media with effusion. *Int J Pediatr Otorhinolaryngol.* Aug 2008;72(8):1215-1223., with permission from Elsevier.

APPENDIX C

COMPARISON OF TEST RESULTS FROM GENERAL ALLERGIST AND ENT ALLERGIST

FIGURES A AND B

Pollens	Prick 1:20	1:100,000	1:10,000	1:1,000
Ash			3	9
Beech			4	
Oak			5	8
Alder				
Birch			6	
Maple Mix	2/10			
Aspen			7	
Cottonwood			8	
Eas Wh. Pine				
Hickory			9	
Black Willow			10	3/1
Elm			11	7/26
Sycamore				
Box Elder			12	3/5
Grass Mix	14/45	@14mins		XXXXX
Sorrel Plantain	3/4			
Lambs Qr Cocklb us Pigweed			13	8/30
Mugwort			14	4/5
Ragweed (S G)			15	3/7
Goldenrod				

Environmental	Prick 1:20	OTHER	Prick 1:20	
Cat pelt	5/20	@19mins		
Cockroach				
Dog	14/45	@14min	16	
Mite D farinae	10/32			
Mite Dpteron				
MOLDS				
Alternaria			17	
Aspergillus			18	
Cladosporium Cur Eak Ru Alx Penula			19	3/14
Epicoccum			20	
Penicilium			21	
Hormodendrum			22	
Other Molds				
Fusarium				
Trichophyton				
Mucor Mix				
Stemphylium				
Helminthsporium				
Latex Prick	1:000	1:100	1:10	Conc

Figure A

ANTIGEN	DILUTION NUMBER						
	7	6	5	4	3	2	1
DUST F							
STD CAT	5	7					
AP DOG			5		5	9	—
DUST F			5		5	5	5
GRASS	7	7/9					
RAGWEED				9	—		
TREE					5	5	7
WEED			5		5	5/9	9
GOLDENROD					5	5	7
INSECT				5	9/9	9	
MOLD A					7	9	
MOLD 5					5	5	
MOLD 10					5	7	
MOLD 15					5	7	
TRICHO					5	7	
Controls					5	6	
NACL							
HISTAMINE						5	
GLYCERIN						11	

Figure B

Comparison of testing results of patient H.F. with chronic middle ear disease as done by both general allergist (top) and ENT allergist (bottom).

PATIENT **H.F.**	GENERAL **Positive by Prick**	GENERAL **Positive by Intradermal**	ENT **Positive by Intradermal**
Dust P			X
Cat	X	X	X
Dog	X		X
Dust F	X		X
Grass			X
Ragweed		X	X
Trees	X	X	X
Weeds	X		X
Goldenrod			X
Cockroach			X
Molds:			X
Alternaria			
Hormodendrum			X
Other Molds			X
Total Positive	**5**	**3**	**17**
Total Tested	**27**	**22**	**17**

Figure A: 27 allergens tested at 1:20 prick plus intradermal, only 5 positive pricks, 3 additional positive by intradermal. Note: No controls noted. Figure B: Intradermal testing by ENT allergist found the same patient positive to all 17 allergens (circled numbers). MISSED by Prick testing: Dust P, Grass, Goldenrod, Cockroach, and all molds.

FIGURES C AND D

Dust	Grass	Ragweed	English Plantain	Weed Mix.	Tree Mix.
1	2	3	4	5	6
O	O	O	O	O	O
Alternaria	**Aspergillus**	**Helminthosporium**	**Cladosporiodes**	**Penicillium**	**Mucor**
7	8	9	10	11	12
O	O	O	O	O	O
Fusarium	**Pullularia**	**Goldenrod**	**Dust Mite Farinae**	**Dust Mite Pter.**	**Pine**
13	14	15	16	17	18
O	O	O	O	O	O
Cat Pelt	**Dog**	**Rabbit**	**Horse**	**Feather**	**Histamine**
19	20				21
O	O				O

Figure C

+ HSthma +   DILUTION NUMBER

ANTIGEN	10	9	8	7	6	5	4	3	2	1
DUST P					5	5	5	5	7	
STD CAT					5	5	5	5	7	
AP DOG					5	5	5	5	7	
DUST F					5	5	5	7	9	
GRASS						5	5	7		
RAGWEED						5	5	7		
TREE						5	7	9		
WEED						5	5	5		
GOLDENROD						5	5	7		
INSECT						5	5	7		
MOLD A							5	7		
MOLD 5							5	5		
MOLD 10					5	7	9	11		
MOLD 15						5	7	9		
TRICHO							5	7		
NACL									5	
HISTAMINE									11	
GLYCERIN									5	

Figure D

Comparison of testing results of patient R.F. with chronic middle ear disease as done by both general allergist (top) and ENT allergist (bottom).

PATIENT H.F.	GENERAL Positive by Prick	GENERAL Positive by Intradermal	ENT Positive by Intradermal
Dust P	X		ˎ X
Cat	X		X
Dog	X		X
Dust F			X
Grass	X		X
Ragweed			X
Trees			X
Weeds	X		
Goldenrod			X
Cockroach			X
Molds:			X
Alternaria			
Hormodendrum			
Other Molds			X
Total Positive	1 positive and 4 questionable		12
Total Tested	17	NONE	12

Figure C: 17 allergens tested at 1:20 prick, none by intradermal; all but one wheal are smaller than or equal to Histamine control. Four borderline positives. MISSED: Most all 17 classes of allergens were below the sensitivity of prick testing. Note: no controls recorded. Figure D: Intradermal testing by ENT allergist found the same patient positive to 15 of 17 allergens (circled numbers). MISSED by Prick testing: Dust F, Grass, Trees, Goldenrod, Cockroach, and molds.

FIGURES E AND F

	PT	ID			PT	ID
NEGATIVE CONTROL						
POSITIVE CONTROL						
DUST AND DANDER (YEAR ROUND)			TREES (continued)			
1. Greer Dust			35. White pine			
2. H.S. Dust			36. Shagbark hickory			
3. A.P. Dust			37. Beech			
4. Mite-Farinae						
5. Mite-Pteronyssinus			MOLDS (YEAR ROUND, SUMMER/FALL)			
6. Cat			38. Alternaria tenuis			
7. Dog			39. Hormodendrum hordei			
8. Cockroach			40. Penicillium mix			
			41. Aspergillus mix			
GRASSES (SPRING/SUMMER)			42. Helminthosporium sativum			
9. Sweet vernal			43. Pullularia pullulans			
10. Blue			44. Curvularia spicifera			
11. Orchard			45. Fusarium solani			
12. Timothy			46. Rhizopus nigricans			
13. Red top			47. Chaetonium globosum			
14. Perennial Rye			48. Mucor mucedo			
			49. Epicoccum purpurascens			
WEEDS (FALL)			50. Cephalosporium acremonium			
15. Ragweed			51. Monilia sitophila			
16. English plantain			52. Phoma betae			
17. Rough pigweed			53. Spondylocladium atrovirens			
18. Lambs quarters			54. Trichoderma viride			
19. Cocklebur			55. Trichophyton mentagrophytes			
20. Goldenrod			56. Candida albicans			
21. Sage						
22. Mugwort			OTHER ANIMALS			
23. Dandelion			57. Horse			
			58. Guinea pig			
TREES (SPRING)			59. Hamster			
24. Cottonwood			60. Rabbit			
25. Black walnut			61. Cat (Bayer AP)			
26. Oak			62. Feather mix			
27. Elm						
28. Sycamore			MISCELLANEOUS			
29. Ash						
30. Box elder						
31. Birch						
32. Maple			received			
33. Tag alder						
34. Quaking aspen						

Figure E

ANTIGEN	DILUTION NUMBER						
	7	6	5	4	3	2	1
DUST P					5	7	7
STD CAT					5	5	7
AP DOG					5	5	5
DUST F					5	5	7
GRASS					5	5	7
RAGWEED				5	7	#4	
TREE					5	5	5
WEED					5	5	7
GOLDENROD					5	5	7
INSECT					5	5	5
MOLD A						7	7
MOLD 5						5	7
MOLD 10						5	7
MOLD 15				5	7	9	
TRICHO						5	7
Controls							
NACl							5
HISTAMINE							9
GLYCERIN							5

Figure F

150

Comparison of testing results of patient P.E. with chronic middle ear disease as done by both general allergist (top) and ENT allergist (bottom).

PATIENT H.F.	GENERAL Positive by Prick	GENERAL Positive by Intradermal		ENT Positive by Intradermal
Dust P				X
Cat	X	X		X
Dog	X			X
Dust F	X			X
Grass				X
Ragweed		X		X
Trees	X	X		X
Weeds	X			X
Goldenrod				X
Cockroach				X
Molds:				X
Alternaria				
Hormodendrum				X
Other Molds				X
Total Positive	5	3		17
Total Tested	27	22		17

Figure E: 28 allergens tested at 1:20 prick, 8 by intradermal. MISSED: All 13 classes of allergens other than Ragweed as all were below the sensitivity of prick testing. Figure F: Intradermal testing by ENT allergist found the same patient positive to 14 of 17 allergens (circled numbers). MISSED by Prick testing: Dust F, Cat, Grass, Weeds, Goldenrod, and all molds.

FIGURES G AND H

	PT	ID		PT	ID
NEGATIVE CONTROL					
POSITIVE CONTROL	+3				
DUST AND DANDER (YEAR ROUND)			TREES (continued)		
1. Greer Dust			35. White pine		
2. H.S. Dust			36. Shagbark hickory		
3. A.P. Dust			37. Beech		
4. Mite-Farinae					
5. Mite-Pteronyssinus			MOLDS (YEAR ROUND, SUMMER/FALL)		
6. Cat			38. Alternaria tenuis		
7. Dog			39. Hormodendrum hordei		
8. Cockroach			40. Penicillium mix		
			41. Aspergillus mix		
GRASSES			42. Helminthosporium sativum		
9. Sweet vernal			43. Pullularia pullulans		
10. Blue			44. Curvularia spicifera		
11. Orchard			45. Fusarium solani		
12. Timothy			46. Rhizopus nigricans		
13. Red top			47. Chaetonium globosum		
14. Perennial Rye			48. Mucor mucedo		
			49. Epicoccum purpurascens		
WEEDS (FALL)			50. Cephalosporium acremonium		
15. Ragweed			51. Monilia sitophila		
16. English plantain			52. Phoma betae		
17. Rough pigweed			53. Spondylocladium atrovirens		
18. Lambs quarters			54. Trichoderma viride		
19. Cocklebur			55. Trichophyton mentagrophytes		
20. Goldenrod			56. Candida albicans		
21. Sage					
22. Mugwort			OTHER ANIMALS		
23. Dandelion			57. Horse		
			58. Guinea pig		
TREES (SPRING)			59. Hamster		
24. Cottonwood			60. Rabbit		
25. Black walnut			61. Cat (Bayer AP)		
26. Oak			62. Feather mix		
27. Elm					
28. Sycamore			MISCELLANEOUS		
29. Ash					
30. Box elder					
31. Birch					
32. Maple					
33. Tag alder					
34. Quaking aspen					

Figure G

DILUTION NUMBER

ANTIGEN	7	6	5	4	3	2
DUST P				5	5	5
STD CAT				5	5	5
AP DOG				5	5	5
DUST F				5	5	7
GRASS				5	5	7
RAGWEED				5	7	7
TREE				5	7	7
WEED				5	5	5
GOLDENROD				5	7	7
INSECT				5	5	7
MOLD A					5	5
MOLD 5					5	5
MOLD 10					5	7
MOLD 15				5	7	7
TRICHO					5	
NACL						5
HISTAMINE						7
GLYCERIN						5

Figure H

Comparison of testing results of patient P.C. with chronic middle ear disease as done by both general allergist (top) and ENT allergist (bottom).

PATIENT H.F.	GENERAL Positive by Prick	GENERAL Positive by Intradermal	ENT Positive by Intradermal
Dust P			
Cat			
Dog			
Dust F		X	X
Grass			X
Ragweed			X
Trees			X
Weeds			
Goldenrod			X
Cockroach			X
Molds:			
Alternaria			
Hormodendrum			X
Other Molds			X
Total Positive	**0**	**1**	**8**
Total Tested	**27**	**0**	**17**

Figure G: 27 allergens were tested at 1:20 prick and all were negative. Five allergens then tested positive by intradermal; all but one wheal are smaller than or equal to Histamine control. MISSED: All 27 classes of allergens were below the sensitivity of prick testing. Figure H: Intradermal testing by ENT allergist found the same patient positive to 8 of 17 allergens (circled numbers). MISSED by Prick testing: Grass, Ragweed, Trees, Goldenrod, Cockroach, and 2 molds.

SOURCES OF GENERAL INFORMATION

WEBSITES

American Academy of Otolaryngic Allergy (AAOA)
www.aaoaf.org

Pan American Allergy Society (PAAS)
www.paas.org

American Academy of Environmental Medicine
www.aaemonline.org

BOOKS

Crook, William G., M.D., and Marjorie Hurt Jones, R.N. *The Yeast Connection Cookbook*. Square One Publishers, 1989.

Rapp, Doris, M.D. *The Impossible Child*. Buffalo, NY: Practical Allergy Research Foundation, 1989.

Thabest Molecular Medicine Inc., 95 E Main Street, Suite 203, Denville, NJ 07834

Clinics of Otolaryngology. *The Role of Allergy in Otitis Media with Effusion*. D. Hurst. July 2011; 44(3).

ABBREVIATIONS

ET = Eustachian tube
OME = Otitis Media with Effusion (or fluid in the middle ear)
IT = Immunotherapy
ENT = Ear, Nose and Throat Surgeon (Otolaryngologist)
IDT = Intradermal Testing

REFERENCES

1. Hurst DS. Allergy management of refractory serous otitis media. *Otolaryngol Head Neck Surg.* Jun 1990;102(6):664-669.

2. Rosenfeld RM, Culpepper L, Doyle KJ, et al. Clinical practice guideline: Otitis media with effusion. *Otolaryngol Head Neck Surg.* May 2004;130(5 Suppl):S95-118.

3. Burton MJ, Krouse JH, Rosenfeld RM. Extracts from The Cochrane Library: Allergen injection immunotherapy for seasonal allergic rhinitis (review). *Otolaryngol Head Neck Surg.* Apr 2007;136(4):511-514.

4. Jacobsen L, Niggemann B, Dreborg S, et al. Specific immunotherapy has long-term preventive effect of seasonal and perennial asthma: 10-year follow-up on the PAT study. *Allergy.* Aug 2007;62(8):943-948.

5. Davila I, Mullol J, Ferrer M, et al. Genetic aspects of allergic rhinitis. *J Investig Allergol Clin Immunol.* 2009;19 Suppl 1:25-31.

6. Alho OP, Koivu M, Sorri M, et al. Risk factors for recurrent acute otitis media and respiratory infection in infancy. *International J Pediatric Otorhinolaryngol.* 1990;19:151-161.

7. Alles R, Parikh A, Hawk L, et al. The prevalence of atopic disorders in children with chronic otitis media with effusion. *Pediatr Allergy Immunol.* Apr 2001;12(2):102-106.

8. Chantzi FM, Kafetzis DA, Bairamis T, et al. IgE sensitization, respiratory allergy symptoms, and heritability independently increase the risk of otitis media with effusion. *Allergy.* Mar 2006;61(3):332-336.

9. Rosenfeld RM, Kay D. Natural history of untreated otitis media. *Laryngoscope.* Oct 2003;113(10):1645-1657.

10. Hurst DS, Venge P. Evidence of eosinophil, neutrophil, and mast-cell mediators in the effusion of OME patients with and without atopy. *Allergy.* May 2000;55(5):435-441.

11. Hurst DS, Venge P. The impact of atopy on neutrophil activity in middle ear effusion from children and adults with chronic otitis media. *Arch Otolaryngol Head Neck Surg.* May 2002;128(5):561-566.

12. Nsouli TM, Nsouli SM, Linde RE, et al. The role of food allergy in serous otitis media. *Annals of Allergy.* 1994;73(3):215-219.

13. Sade J, Wolfson S, Sachs Z, et al. The infant's eustachian tube lumen: the pharyngeal part. *J Laryngol Otol.* 1986;100:129-134.

14. Straetemans M, van Heerbeek N, Schilder AG, et al. Eustachian tube function before recurrence of otitis media with effusion. *Arch Otolaryngol Head Neck Surg.* Feb 2005;131(2):118-123.

15. O'Reilly RC, He Z, Bloedon E, et al. The role of extraesophageal reflux in otitis media in infants and children. *Laryngoscope.* Jul 2008;118(7 Part 2 Suppl 116):1-9.

16. Derebery MJ. Allergic management of Meniere's disease: an outcome study. *Otolaryngol Head Neck Surg.* Feb 2000;122(2):174-182.

17. McKay SP, Meslemani D, Stachler RJ, et al. Intradermal positivity after negative prick testing for inhalants. *Otolaryngol Head Neck Surg.* Aug 2006;135(2):232-235.

18. Gordon BR. Allergy skin tests for inhalants and foods: Comparison of methods in common use. *Otol Clin NA.* Vol 31; 1998:35-54.

19. Hurst DS, Gordon BR, Fornadley JA, et al. Safety of home-based and office allergy immunotherapy: A multicenter prospective study. *Otolaryngol Head Neck Surg.* Nov 1999;121(5):553-561.

20. Ali M, Ramanarayanan M. A computerized micro-ELISA assay for allergen-specific antibodies. *American J Clinic Path.* 1984;81:591-601.

21. Hurst DS. Efficacy of allergy immunotherapy as a treatment for patients with chronic otitis media with effusion. *Int J Pediatr Otorhinolaryngol.* Aug 2008;72(8):1215-1223.

22. Taskinen TM, Laitinen S, Nevalainen A, et al. Immunoglobulin G antibodies to moulds in school-children from moisture problem schools. *Allergy.* Jan 2002;57(1):9-16.

23. Hurst DS. The association of otitis media with effusion and allergy as demonstrated by intradermal skin testing and eosinophil cationic protein levels in both middle ear effusions and mucosal biopsies. *Laryngoscope.* 1996;106:1128-1137.

24. Balatsouras DG, Eliopoulos P, Rallis E, et al. Improvement of otitis media with effusion after treatment of asthma with leukotriene antagonists in children with co-existing disease. *Drugs Exp Clin Res.* 2005;31 Suppl:7-10.

25. Bousquet J, Cabrera P, Berkman N, et al. The effect of treatment with omalizumab, an anti-IgE antibody, on asthma exacerbations and emergency medical visits in patients with severe persistent asthma. *Allergy.* Mar 2005;60(3):302-308.

26. Ernst E. Chiropractic manipulation for non-spinal pain--a systematic review. *N Z Med J.* Aug 8 2003;116(1179):U539.

27. Passalacqua G, Canonica GW. Long-lasting clinical efficacy of allergen specific immunotherapy. *Allergy.* Apr 2002;57(4):275-276.

28. Francis JN, James LK, Paraskevopoulos G, et al. Grass pollen immunotherapy: IL-10 induction and suppression of late responses precedes IgG4 inhibitory antibody activity. *J Allergy Clin Immunol.* May 2008;121(5):1120-1125 e1122.

29. Bousquet J, Van Cauwenberge P, Khaltaev N. Allergic rhinitis and its impact on asthma. *J Allergy Clin Immunol.* Nov 2001;108(5 Suppl):S147-334.

30. Johansson SG, Bieber T, Dahl R, et al. Revised nomenclature for allergy for global use: Report of the Nomenclature Review Committee of the World Allergy Organization, October 2003. *J Allergy Clin Immunol.* May 2004;113(5):832-836.

31. Mosmann TR, Cherwinski H, Bond MW, et al. Two types of murine helper T cell clone. I. Definition according to profiles of lymphokine activities and secreted proteins. *J Immunol.* Apr 1 1986;136(7):2348-2357.

32. Hurst DS, Amin K, Sevéus L, et al. Evidence of mast cell activity in the middle ear of children with otitis media with effusion. *Laryngoscope.* 1999;109:471-477.

33. Wright ED, Hurst D, Miotto D, et al. Increased expression of major basic protein (MBP) and interleukin-5(IL-5) in middle ear biopsy specimens from atopic patients with persistent otitis media with effusion. *Otolaryngol Head Neck Surg.* Nov 2000;123(5):533-538.

34. Hurst DS, Ramanarayanan MP, Weekley M. Evidence of possible localized specific IgE production in middle ear fluid as demonstrated by ELISA testing. *Otolaryngol Head Neck Surg.* 1999;121:224-230.

35. Labadie RF, Jewett BS, Hart CF, et al. Allergy increases susceptibility to otitis media with effusion in a rat model. Second place--Resident Clinical Science Award 1998. *Otolaryngol Head Neck Surg.* Dec 1999;121(6):687-692.

36. Palva T, Hayry P, Yikoski J. Lymphocyte morphology in middle ear effusions. *Ann Otol Rhinol Laryngol.* 1980;89 (Suppl 68):143-146.

37. Hamilos D, Leung D, Wood R, et al. Evidence for distinct cytokine expression in allergic versus nonallergic chronic sinusitis. *J Allergy Clin Immunol.* 1995;96:537-544.

38. Egan RW, Umland SP, Cuss RM, et al. Biology of interleukin-5 and its relevance to allergic disease. *Allergy.* 1996;51:71-81.

39. Bikhazi P, Ryan AF. Expression of immunoregulatory cytokines during acute and chronic middle ear immune response. *Laryngoscope.* 1995;105:629-634.

40. Hurst DS. *The middle ear: The inflammatory response in children with otitis media with effusion and the impact of atopy. Clinical and histochemical studies.* [PhD]. Uppsala, Sweden: Comprehensive Summaries of Uppsala Dessertations from the Faculty of Medicine, Dept of Immunology and Clincal Chemistry #978, Uppsala University, Sweden; 2000.

41. Jang CH, Kim YH. Demonstration of RANTES and eosinophilic cataionic protein in otitis media with effusion with allergy. *Int J Pediatr Otorhinolaryngol.* May 2003;67(5):531-533.

42. Nguyen LH, Manoukian JJ, Sobol SE, et al. Similar allergic inflammation in the middle ear and the upper airway: evidence linking otitis media with effusion to the united airways concept. *J Allergy Clin Immunol.* Nov 2004;114(5):1110-1115.

43. Lasisi AO, Arinola OG, Olayemi O. Role of elevated immunoglobulin E levels in suppurative otitis media. *Ann Trop Paediatr.* Jun 2008;28(2):123-127.

44. Sobol SE, Taha R, Schloss MD, et al. T(H)2 cytokine expression in atopic children with otitis media with effusion. *J Allergy Clin Immunol.* Jul 2002;110(1):125-130.

45. Stenstrom C, Ingvarsson L. General illness and need of medical care in otitis prone children. *Int J Pediatr Otorhinolaryngol.* Mar 1994;29(1):23-32.

46. Lazo-Saenz JG, Galvan-Aguilera AA, Martinez-Ordaz VA, et al. Eustachian tube dysfunction in allergic rhinitis. *Otolaryngol Head Neck Surg.* Apr 2005;132(4):626-629.

47. Doner F, Yariktas M, Demirci M. The role of allergy in recurrent otitis media with effusion. *J Investig Allergol Clin Immunol.* 2004;14(2):154-158.

48. Bluestone CD. Eustachian tube function and allergy in otitis media. *Pediatrics.* 1978;61(5):753-760.

49. Skoner D, Gentile D, Mandel E, et al. Otitis Media. In: Adkinson N, B Bochner B, J Yunginger J, et al., eds. *Middleton's Allergy Principles & Practice.* Vol 2. 6th ed. Philadelphia: Mosby, Inc; 2003:1437-1454.

50. Lieberman P, Blaiss M. Allergic Diseases of the Eye and Ear. In: Leslie Grammer PG, ed. *Patterson's Allergic Diseases.* 6th ed. Philadelphia, Pa: Lippincott Williams & Wilkins; 2002:209-223.

51. Tewfik TL, Mazer B. The links between allergy and otitis media with effusion. *Curr Opin Otolaryngol Head Neck Surg.* Jun 2006;14(3):187-190.

52. Friedman RA, Doyle WJ, Casselbrant ML, et al. Immunologic-mediated eustachian tube obstruction: A double-blind crossover study. *J Allergy and Clin Immunol.* 1983;71:442-447.

53. Ackerman M, Friedman R, Doyle W, et al. Antigen-induced eustachian tube obstruction: an internasal provocative challenge test. *J Allergy Clin Immunol.* 1984;73:604-609.

54. Bernstein J. Recent advances in immunologic reactivity in otitis media with effusion. *J Allergy Clin. Immunol.* 1988;81:1004-1009.

55. Doyle W, Friedman R, Fireman P. Eustachian tube obstruction in passively sensitized rhesus monkeys following provocative nasal antigen challenge. *Arch Otolaryngol.* 1984;110:508-511.

56. Takahashi H, Hayashi M, Sato H, et al. Primary deficits in eustachian tube function in patients with otitis media with effusion. *Arch Otolaryngol Head Neck Surg.* 1989;115:581-584.

57. Hardy SM, Heavner SB, White DR, et al. Late-phase allergy and eustachian tube dysfunction. *Otolaryngol Head Neck Surg.* Oct 2001;125(4):339-345.

58. Braunstahl GJ, Overbeek SE, Kleinjan A, et al. Nasal allergen provocation induces adhesion molecule expression and tissue eosinophilia in upper and lower airways. *J Allergy Clin Immunol.* Mar 2001;107(3):469-476.

59. Ohashi Y, Nakai Y, Tanaka A, et al. Soluble adhesion molecules in middle ear effusions from patients with chronic otitis media with effusion. *Clin Otolaryngol.* 1998;23:231-234.

60. Ebmeyer J, Furukawa M, Pak K, et al. Role of mast cells in otitis media. *J Allergy Clin Immunol.* Nov 2005;116(5):1129-1135.

61. Iino Y, Kakizaki K, Katano H, et al. Eosinophil chemoattractants in the middle ear of patients with eosinophilic otitis media. *Clin Exp Allergy.* Oct 2005;35(10):1370-1376.

62. Smirnova MG, Birchall JP, Pearson JP. The immunoregulatory and allergy-associated cytokines in the aetiology of the otitis media with effusion. *Mediators Inflamm.* Apr 2004;13(2):75-88.

63. McKenna M. Otitis Media. In: Bailey B, Johnson J, Newlands S, et al., eds. *Head and Neck Surgery—Otolaryngology.* Vol 1: Lippincott Williams & Wilkins; 1998, 2006.

64. Chinoy B, Yee E, Bahna SL. Skin testing versus radioallergosorbent testing for indoor allergens. *Clin Mol Allergy.* Apr 15 2005;3(1):4.

65. Bernstein JM, Ellis E, Li P. The Role of IgE-mediated Hypersensitivity in Otitis Media With Effusion. *Otolaryngol Head and Neck Surg.* 1981;89:874.

66. Johansson SGO. The development and clinical significance of the Radioallergosorbent test. In: Fadal R, Nalebuff D, eds. *RAST in Clinical Allergy*: Symposia Foundation; 1989:25-33.

67. Dohlman FG. Allergiska Processer i Mellanorat. *Nord. med. tidskr.* 1943;20:2231.

68. Mao C-Y. Allergy as a contributing factor to biologic deafness. *Arch Otolaryngol.* 1942;35:582-586.

69. Jordan R. Chronic secretory otitis media. *Laryngoscope.* 1949;59(Sept):1002-1015.

70. Solow IA. Is serous otitis media due to allergy or infection? *Ann Allergy.* 1958;16:297-299.

71. Lecks HL. Allergic aspects of serous otitis media in childhood. *NY State J Med.* 1961;61:2737-2743.

72. Fernandez A, McGovern J. Secretory otitis media in allergic infants and children. *Southern Medical Journal.* 1965;58:581-586.

73. Whitcomb NJ. Allergy therapy in serous otitis media associated with allergic rhinitis. *Annals of Allergy.* 1965;23:232-236.

74. Draper WL. Secretory otitis media in children: a study of 540 children. *Laryngoscope.* 1967(77):636-653.

75. Hall LJ, Lukat RM. Results of allergy treatment on the Eustachian tube in chronic serous otitis media. *Am J Otol.* Oct 1981;3(2):116-121.

76. McMahan JT, Calenoff E, Croft DJ, et al. Chronic otitis media with effusion and allergy: modified RAST analysis of 119 cases. *Otolaryngol Head Neck Surg.* May-Jun 1981;89(3 Pt 1):427-431.

77. Sanz M, Tabar A, Manrique M, et al. Local serum IgE in patients affected by otitis media with effusion. *Allergol et immunopathol.* 1986;14:483-487.

78. Tomonaga K, Kurono Y, Moge G. The role of nasal allergy in otitis media with effusion, a clinical study. *Acta Otolaryngol.* 1988;458(Suppl):41-47.

79. Becker S, Koch T, Philipp A. Allergic origin of recurrent middle ear effusion and adenoids in young children[German]. *HNO-Klinik, Medizinischen Hochschule Hannover.* 1991;39:122-124.

80. Corey J, Adham R, Abbass A, et al. The role of IgE-mediated hypersensitivity in otitis media with effusion. *Amer J Otolaryngol.* 1994;15:138-144.

81. Psifidis A, Hatzistilianou M, Samaras K, et al. Atopy and otitis media in children. Paper presented at: Proceedings of the 7th International Congress of Pediatric Otorhinolaryngology, 1998; Helsinki, Finland.

82. Lasisi AO, Arinola OG, Bakare RA. Serum and middle ear immunoglobulins in suppurative otitis media. *ORL J Otorhinolaryngol Relat Spec.* 2008;70(6):389-392.

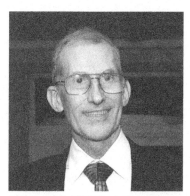

ABOUT THE AUTHOR

Dr. Hurst has been in private practice in Maine for 35 years since having completed his residency at Tufts University where he continues to partici-pate on the teaching staff. He earned his PhD in clinical immunology at Uppsala University, Sweden. He has published 18 articles on chronic middle ear disease and is on the editorial review boards of most major journals in his field, including: *Laryngoscope, Allergy, International Journal of Pedia-triac Otorhinolaryngology, Archives of Otolaryngology, and Otolaryngology-Head and Neck Surgery*. Dr. Hurst has presented instruction courses on the relation of allergy to chronic ear disease each of the past 20 years at the annual meetings of the American Academy of Otolaryngology-Head and Neck Surgery and/or the American Academy of Otolaryngologic Allergy. Having practiced the entire range of Ear, Nose and Throat surgery Dr. Hurst now devotes his full time to allergy as it impacts upper respiratory diseases.

CPSIA information can be obtained at www.ICGtesting.com
Printed In the USA
BVOW06s1740140216

436689BV00013B/144/P